# ARE WE
# SCARING
# OURSELVES
# TO DEATH?

# H. AARON COHL

# ARE WE SCARING OURSELVES TO DEATH?

HOW PESSIMISM, PARANOIA, AND A MISGUIDED
MEDIA ARE LEADING US TOWARD DISASTER

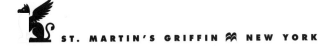

ST. MARTIN'S GRIFFIN ❧ NEW YORK

Another book by
AFFINITY COMMUNICATIONS CORP.

# DISCLAIMER

This book is meant entirely and solely for entertainment purposes, and to urge you to question what you read and hear reported by the media (as well as what you read in this book!). This publication must not be mistaken for a book that provides detailed and/or technical medical, nutritional, financial, scientific, or legal information and advice. The creator of this book is not engaged in rendering medical, nutritional, financial, scientific, or legal information, advice or other professional service. If medical, nutritional, financial, scientific, or legal information, advice, or other expert assistance is required, the  services of a competent professional should be sought.

A THOMAS DUNNE BOOK.

An imprint of St. Martin's Press.

Are We Scaring Ourselves to Death?

*Production Editor: David Stanford Burr*

Library of Congress Cataloging-in-Publication Data

Cohl, H. Aaron.
    Are we scaring ourselves to death? / H. Aaron Cohl.—1st St.
Martin's Griffin ed.
        p. cm.
    "A Thomas Dunne book"—T.p. verso.
    ISBN 0-312-15056-3
    1. Mass media—United States—Psychological aspects. 2. Social
psychology—United States. 3. Risk perception—United States.
4. Risk communication—United States. 5. Sensationalism in
journalism—United States. I. Title.
HN90.M3C64     1997
302—dc20                                         96-38570
                                                 CIP

First St. Martin's Griffin Edition: April 1997

10  9  8  7  6  5  4  3  2  1

C O N T E N T S

PREFACE                                                    1

## INTRODUCTION

HOW WE SCARE OURSELVES TO DEATH                            7
MEDIA MADNESS                                             12
TECHNOLOGY: A DOUBLE-EDGED SWORD                          19
HUMAN PSYCHOLOGY IN THE MODERN AGE                        24

## TO YOUR HEALTH!

HEALTHY, WEALTHY, AND WISE (?)                            31
BREAST CANCER SCARE                                       34
AMPLE ENDOWMENT: THE PUMPED-UP HYSTERIA
   OVER BREAST IMPLANTS                                   38
AN APPLE A DAY . . .                                      42
SOUR GRAPES                                               45
FEAR OF FAT                                               47
AIDS, FEAR, AND THE MIDDLE-CLASS HETEROSEXUAL             50
THE SCARLET "H"                                           53
EVERYTHING CAUSES CANCER                                  57
"PESTICIDES PREVENT CANCER" (NO, THAT'S NOT A TYPO)       60
HAMBURGERS: THE ALL-AMERICAN . . . POISON?                65
MAD AS A . . . COW?!?                                     67
NIGHT OF THE LIVING FLESH-EATING SLIME . . .              70

HAUNTED BY HANTA                                                      73
JUST A SMOKE SCREEN?                                                  75

## HOME SWEET HOME?

THERE'S NO PLACE LIKE HOME                                           81
RADIOACTIVE DISHES? RADON IN THE HOME                                82
LEAD-BASED PAINT: DANGER IN YOUR OWN HOME                            85
ASBESTOS EVERYWHERE                                                  87
WILL VIDEO DISPLAY TERMINALS MAKE YOU "TERMINAL"?                    90
BIOTECHNOLOGY FOR BREAKFAST: SUPER-COW OR COW VILLAIN?              92

## URBAN/SUBURBAN SURVIVAL

THE SAFE MEAN STREETS                                                97
YOUR HOME IS YOUR FORTRESS                                           99
ROAD WARRIORS                                                       102
A CALL TO ARMS                                                      106
WORK CAN KILL YOU: DEATH ON THE JOB                                 109
FEAR OF FLYING                                                      112

## OUR ENVIRONMENT

THE GREEN MONSTER                                                   119
THE GREENHOUSE EFFECT: A STORY OF HOT AIR?                          121
"THE SKY IS FALLING!"                                               125
DEATH BY DIOXIN?                                                    128
ELECTROMAGNETIC FIELDS: A FIELD OF DREAMS?                          131
NUKING THE MUSHROOM CLOUD OF FEAR                                   134
GO FISH                                                             138
THE SPERM, THE EGG, AND THE INDUSTRIAL REVOLUTION                   141

## CONCLUSION

WHO LOSES? WHO WINS?                                                147

# ACKNOWLEDGMENT

This book would not have been possible without the extraordinary efforts of a select few. Thank you, Cherilyn Parsons, for your diligent research and writing. And thank you, also, Jordan Lewis and Thora Christiansen, for pinch-hitting during crunch time.

# PREFACE

I t's 8:00 in the morning. You shout at your children to hurry up and brush their teeth after breakfast. They use fluoride toothpaste, of course. They've just finished eating breakfast: granola that you made from scratch because the store-bought version has so many additives. Those ingredient lists with their long names are so overwhelming that you've decided they're just not worth deciphering, even though store-bought cereal is a lot less expensive. The kids eat their granola with milk that you purchased at a health food store because the cows that produce that milk were not injected with bovine growth hormone. The non-BGH milk is twice as expensive, but your kids are worth it. It's too bad your food bills are so high that you've had to take on a second job and can't spend as much time with your family as you'd like.

The kids run down the stairs to get in the car. You notice that the carpet runner is slippery, and you've read that more people are hurt from simple mishaps around the house on stairs, in the kitchen, or in the bathroom than in more attention-getting though unusual accidents. But what can you do? You can't afford a new carpet runner right now, much less a new house without stairs. You grab the kids' lunches — no apples or other fruit, thanks to pesticides — just peanut-butter-and-jelly sandwiches on wheat bread. But this too makes you nervous because you heard last week on the news that peanut butter can cause cancer. You set the house alarm and lock the door carefully, recalling that a house five blocks away was burglarized last week.

You strap the kids into the car with seat belts. The elementary school is only a fifteen-minute walk, but crime has increased so much that you hardly dare let them outside alone. Only last month, a seven-year-old girl was abducted from a town on the other side of the state. As you pull out of the driveway, you notice tire marks on your neighbor's lawn. More vandalism? It seems that even the suburbs are no longer safe. Or maybe it was just their sixteen-year-old learning how to back out of the driveway.

You're on the alert as you drive. Drunk drivers are a real menace. There's a beat-up car behind you. Instinctively you press the switch that automatically locks all the car doors. You check the gas gauge; yes, you have enough gas to outrun them if they pull a gun. You remember that you needed to stop at the ATM for money, but in your rush you forgot your ATM card. The money will have to wait.

It's a beautiful sunny day. You wish you'd had the kids put on sunblock. The ozone layer is becoming so thin, the news said, that just being out in the sun is enough to cause skin cancer. Maybe you can bring sunblock to the school later, during your lunch break at work. But then, you hate to drive so much. All that pollution from car exhaust is really killing the atmosphere.

You reach into your purse for a Tylenol. God, you have a headache already. The pill comes in a foil-sealed plastic bottle, which itself comes in a sealed box. You're glad they take such precautions against tampering.

The kids are fiddling with their lunch bags in the backseat — you never let them ride in the passenger seat in the front, which is known as the "death seat" in car accidents. They're complaining about the peanut-butter-and-jelly sandwiches. "Can we go out for hamburgers for dinner?" they wail.

Of course not! Don't they remember how four children died after eating contaminated hamburgers in the northwest United States in 1993? You'll make some sort of dinner later. If you cook chicken long enough, you should be able to kill any bacteria that might harm your children. You'd never serve them fish — not with all the poisons you've heard about in seafood. How about beef? Well, if it won't give them mad cow disease, it will clog their arteries so badly they'll have a heart attack before they're twenty years old. You wish you could serve vegetarian foods like tofu, but the tofu at the health food store sits in water, and you've read reports that dangerous bacteria breed in water like that. Some scientists on the news argue that food should be "irradiated" to kill all the bacteria in meat, fruit, vegetables, and milk that cause hundreds of deaths per year. You think these scientists are crazy. Do they want to give us *more* radiation in our world? More cancer?

That reminds you to visit your Aunt Beatrice in the hospital later that evening. She has cancer. Yes, she smoked for a few years, but she's sure she got cancer from asbestos in her house. It was an old place, and it was shaken up a bit from the last earthquake. Come to think of it, her grandchildren are a bit strange — a little slow, it seems. They spent last summer with Beatrice, the summer after the earthquake. You're sure that she doesn't know about the dangers of lead-based paint, but her house is probably full of it. Lead-based paint can cause neurological damage.

You turn on the radio to hear some news and drown out the kids in the backseat. The newscaster reports the alarming results of a recent study that shows that breast implants can cause cancer. You're glad you never had implants. Who cares if you're a bit flat-chested? But your cousin's daughter wants to be a fashion model, and she got implants. Yes, she looks great, but she'll die young. . . . You mentally slap yourself for feeling vindicated. And then you realize how chilling it must be for all those young women to hear news reports saying that their implants might cause their death.

Speaking of which: You have to remember to cancel the mammogram you scheduled for next week. You just don't want all that radiation from the X ray coursing through your body. You'll take your chances, thank you.

You reach the kids' school and carefully eye the other children. Do any of them have AIDS? Doesn't look like it. Thank God you're married. Heterosexuals are dropping like flies from AIDS.

Your kids unlatch their seat belts and jump out. You call to them, "Don't play outside today, okay?" The news also reported a first-stage smog alert. They wave. You make a mental note to rent a video later so that they won't go outside after school. But it's so hard these days to find a video that doesn't promote violence. You'd never let them just turn on the TV — all that smut! And even when you do let them watch TV — a movie you've rented — they have to sit far from the set to avoid those cancer-causing electromagnetic rays coming from the screen. You don't want them to end up like Beatrice. But then, which risk is greater — watching TV (smut, violence, and electromagnetic radiation), or playing outside (crime, smog, and possibly contagious playmates)?

You shout to your kids the final words that you say every single day: "Be careful. . . ."

Be careful . . . be careful . . . be careful . . .

# INTRODUCTION

# HOW WE SCARE OURSELVES TO DEATH

*"The world is coming to an end in our lifetime!"*
*"Disaster is about to strike!"*
*"The sky is falling! The sky is falling!"*
*"Birth defects on the rampage!"*
*"Besieged by murder, rape, and robbery!"*
*"Hamburgers kill kids!"*

Are these the pronouncements of wild-eyed, crazy preachers on street corners — and the Chicken Littles of fairy tales? Are they headlines from tabloids sold at supermarket check-out stands? No — these types of headlines appear in respectable media such as the *New York Times*, the *Los Angeles Times*, the *Chicago Tribune*, *Time*, *Newsweek*, and the evening network news.

What do we do when these sources tell us that we're not very safe in our own homes? That it's hardly safe to venture *out* of our homes, thanks to drive-by shootings, ATM holdups, and workplace violence? That the food we eat will give us cancer? That the air we breathe will give us cancer? That practically everything gives us cancer? How about when national news magazines imply that our heterosexual, longtime lover could give us AIDS?

What do we think when we see famous research scientists disagreeing in public about whether our world will enter a new ice age due to a "greenhouse effect" — or whether the ozone layer is really thinning or not? What do we do each morning when one day a scientific study tells us not to drink coffee (caffeine is dangerous) and then the next day another study tells us that caffeine helps our memory and attention? What do we do each evening when scientists tell us that red wine is bad for us, and that mineral water is good — and then a couple of months later, red wine is shown to help prevent heart disease, and mineral water (Perrier) is found to be contaminated? What *do* we pour into our glasses for dinner?

We become paralyzed with fear and unable to separate the real risks from the exaggerated ones. We can become so overwhelmed by the "risks" of modern society that we make poor choices in avoiding risks:

- For example, we fear radiation, which is known to cause cancer (as the media relentlessly tell us). Therefore, when it comes time to have a mammogram, a woman refuses because she fears the radiation exposure of the X ray. However, the risk of the radiation dose is minuscule compared to the benefits of finding a cancerous breast tumor before it becomes life-threatening. This woman quite literally could be scaring herself to death.
- A heterosexual man could be so nervous about contracting AIDS heterosexually — a tiny, tiny risk — that he never dates anyone and never marries. To avoid the minimal risk of contracting AIDS, he experiences the far greater health risk of remaining single. Many studies have shown that single men experience more depression and poorer health than do married men.
- A teenage girl is frightened by the stories she reads in magazines about pesticides on fruits and vegetables. Therefore, she stops eating fruits and vegetables, even though the pesticide risk is very small and deemed safe by the federal government. Soon she develops many nutritional imbalances and damages her internal organs. All this comes from not eating fruits and vegetables — the healthiest, most nutrition-packed foods available — thanks to her excessive fears of media-hyped pesticides.

Our society has become so focused on risks and fears that we really are scaring ourselves to death.

Each day the media bombard us with frightening statistics that reach into every corner of our lives. Crime rates are rising, the "authorities" warn us. No neighborhood is safe. Local newspapers land on our doorsteps alerting us to the atrocities committed daily in our own communities. We are vulnerable to attack even in our cars as we negotiate the increasingly congested highways (complete with freeway shootings) on our way to school and work (where we might face random killings, as in the recent post-office shootings). Assuming we get through the day unscathed and decide to treat ourselves to a movie, we are met with alarming reports about the life-threatening fat content of even the unbuttered popcorn at the local Cineplex.

But is urban living in the 1990s really more dangerous than life in the '70s, or even the '50s? Are we scaring ourselves to death for good reason, or are we responding to "prompts" by special interest groups with hidden agendas, or, more probably, by the media, who know that catastrophes sell better than "all-is-well" headlines?

The truth is, you're safer than you think. Life is far safer today than twenty years ago. We live in the safest, most healthful civilization in the history of the planet. Here's a preview of a few "scares" we will explore in this book.

## CRIME

Crime has dropped 25 percent, not increased, in the last twenty years. Data drawn from the Federal Bureau of Investigation indicate that more than 90 percent of all Americans are safer today than they were two decades ago. Murder is not at an all-time high. The end of Prohibition in 1933 saw murder at its highest per capita level in this century, and that was before violent movies and video games. Murder rates in the late-nineteenth-century days of the Wild West were far higher still.

The fact is that many of the "facts" you know about crime are actually exaggerated, taken out of context, or sometimes just plain wrong. You can sleep easier tonight once you know the real story!

## HEALTH

We've never been healthier — nor so worried about our health.

Cancer is on the increase. That's true. We all see family and friends dying of this horrible disease. However, cancer is increasing for two reasons that are actually very positive to our health. First, medical technology has advanced so far that we live a lot longer than before (250 percent longer than in the early 1900s!). We don't die from other causes, such as tuberculosis and influenza, which killed our forefathers and mothers. Second, doctors can now diagnose cancer more easily because they have more sophisticated diagnostic tools and also because we are better educated about the importance of early cancer detection.

Is secondhand smoke really a killer? For once the cigarette companies may be right that the threat to normal healthy adults is exaggerated. Secondhand smoke does carry some danger, but only if you breathe huge and dense quantities of it for long periods. We're overly frightened of an infrequent whiff of cigarette smoke.

How about the much-maligned pesticides? We will show that the use of pesticides actually helps *prevent* cancer — by increasing the supply of healthful, affordable fruits and vegetables.

## HOME SWEET HOME

It's true that there are killers lurking in our homes. These include buckets (fifty children annually are killed by drowning in buckets), swimming pools (six hundred Americans die annually by drowning in pools), bathtubs, staircases, and so forth.

But the risks we hear about include electromagnetic radiation emitted from power lines near our houses — which has never been proven to cause cancer. We hear about the dangers of household cleaning chemicals. But lye, the chemical used to make soap on the American frontier, was more caustic and dangerous than our modern household cleaning products, which come in spray-top bottles (so we don't have to touch the chemical) or with child-proof caps.

We hear about the terrible results of exposure to lead-based paint. But modern regulations banned lead-based paint over twenty years ago, and licensed contractors exist specifically to remove such paint from older houses.

How about the dangers of exposure to asbestos? Stop worrying. The only way you're likely to develop lung cancer from asbestos is if the insulation in an older home or building is shaken loose in an earthquake, for example, and you remain inside for an extended period of time, breathing in the fibers. You also can develop asbestos problems if you live in a truly dilapidated house with disintegrating asbestos insulation. Thankfully, this doesn't describe the conditions in which most of us live.

## OUR ENVIRONMENT

If you listen closely to environmental groups, which often have the sympathy of the news media, you'll soon believe that we as a species will be extinct in a hundred years (if not sooner). We'll have no forests left after decades of thoughtless clear-cutting. Thanks to the greenhouse effect (created by automobiles and industrial pollution), our atmosphere will have heated up so much that the fertile Midwest will be a desert, and California will be under the Pacific Ocean. The ozone layer will be only a fond memory. Ultraviolet rays from the sun will blast what's left of the earth with cancer-causing radiation. But that won't really matter because all the fish will already have been killed by dioxin emissions from industrial plants. Other species will also be extinct.

Of course, none of this is likely to occur because we will already have blown ourselves up with nuclear bombs. Or the nuclear power plants that we built around the world will have melted down, releasing so much radioactive waste that all life will have become extinct anyway, dying of horrible, slow, painful diseases.

Now if *that* doesn't scare you to death, nothing will. *However* — yes, we can say a big "however" — pay attention to these facts:

Our water and soil have become cleaner, not dirtier, over the past twenty years. We're increasing the percentage of protected forests in our nation, and we're slowing the destruction of rain forests in Third World countries. We're dramatically cutting down on carbon dioxide and lead emissions from petroleum fuels. For example, automobiles today emit only 1 percent of the pollution that spewed from the exhaust pipes of cars in the 1970s. Smog is declining around the country. Manufacturing of chlorofluorocarbons (CFCs), the alleged culprit in thinning our planet's ozone layer, stopped completely in 1995. Species that were once "endangered" are now proliferating. We can swim again in the Great Lakes, Puget Sound, and the Chesapeake Bay. The national recycling rate is about 22 percent, seven times the rate only ten years ago (*USA Weekend*, 14–16 April 1995). Nuclear energy could lessen our dependence on foreign oil — and reduce petroleum pollution even further. The use of fiber-optic cable means that we need to mine less copper to "wire" the nation.

The environment is getting better — thanks to the activism of concerned citizens and government. Now we can take a deep breath (of cleaner air) and relax a bit, confident in the safeguards that we have put in place.

## SO WHY ARE WE SCARING OURSELVES TO DEATH?

If everything is so much better than it was twenty years ago, much less a hundred years ago, why do we hear about more risks than ever before? Why are we so scared? The next three chapters give some insight into *why* we're scaring ourselves to death, in spite of all the good news. You'll learn how to moderate your own fears so you can live a happier — and, yes, *healthier* — life.

# MEDIA MADNESS

"What constitutes news is not necessarily what constitutes a significant public health problem," says John Graham, Director of the Center for Risk Analysis at the Harvard School of Public Health. "The bizarre, the mysterious, that which people have difficulty imagining happening"—that's news, that's what the media cover.
                                        —David Shaw, *Los Angeles Times,* 12 September 1994

A *Boston Globe* reporter recounts how she managed to get her article about the ozone layer on the front page of her newspaper. This reporter had learned from a Harvard University scientist that there was "a very high probability" of a large hole developing by the year 2000. She wanted this story to make a big splash, both for the newspaper and her own career. However, her editor said that the story would only appear on page one if the Harvard scientist said that there would *definitely* be a large ozone hole.

The reporter went back to the scientist. Would it be possible to stretch his assertion, just a bit? As the reporter said, she "negotiated something that really wasn't accurate . . . something much bolder than what was true." (Sometimes scientists aren't adverse to exaggeration; they want publicity, too.) The outcome? Her story ran on the front page. The public read in a respectable, reliable newspaper that a hole in the ozone layer would appear before the end of the century.

This story, related by David Shaw in the *Los Angeles Times* (13 September 1994), illustrates only one of the many pitfalls of media reporting today: that journalists can distort a story for their own motives. The result can be that the public becomes unnecessarily alarmed.

Many of us aren't aware of the limitations and biases of the news media. If the *Boston Globe* reports it — or the *New York Times*, or the network news, or a national news weekly — it must be true, at least for the most part, right?

Yes, *for the most part*. And certainly the media have given extremely useful warnings to the public — for example, about the dangers of the Dalkon Shield, Ford Pinto, and high-fat foods. On the other hand, the media also contribute to scaring us to death. In our age of sound bites, sensationalism, "packaging" of people and concepts, and multiplicity of media forms, we must become "media literate," to use the phrase of an organization called the Center for Media Literacy. This chapter will explore the ways in which the media contribute to scare stories.

### FRONT-PAGE FEVER

Garnering the front-page story, or the "top of the news" on television, is a coup for a journalist. A reporter can overplay a story to grab the attention of an editor and the public.

If we're honest, we'll admit that we're all tempted to exaggerate occasionally for effect. Other times an issue is so complicated that we find ourselves skipping to the really interesting parts to explain it to someone else. Or we face a tight deadline that means cutting corners on "the whole truth."

The people who write and edit newspapers, magazines, and television shows are no different than we are. It's just that millions of people listen to what they say. That gives their little exaggerations and errors a large impact.

### JOURNALISTS AREN'T SCIENTISTS

Journalists don't have microscopes at their desks or PhD diplomas on their walls. Most journalists, even those who cover exclusively science, medicine, or the environment, don't have training in assessing scientific validity. It takes years of training and experience to evaluate scientific methodology, shortcomings, caveats, and so forth. Journalists aren't scientific experts. Rather, they are trained to gather material and investigate, dissect, or summarize it to present the story clearly (and sometimes entertainingly, especially in television news) to the public. Their task of sorting the real science from the pseudoscience is made even more difficult because there are often conflicting research studies on the same topic.

Nevertheless, we trust journalists to sort through the science and give us "truth." We trust them to tell us which scientists are quacks and which are reliable. Sometimes they just don't come through for us. If a media-savvy quack claims to have found a cure for AIDS, or (worse) claims that AIDS can be transmitted by, say, holding hands, a journalist might report such a "finding" to the public — even though no other scientists have validated the conclusions, and the methodology is wrong.

## THE COMPLICATIONS OF SIMPLIFICATION

Another way that the media tend to scare us to death is by oversimplifying risks. Virtually all the health and environmental risks that we hear about are extremely complex, but how can a journalist communicate those complexities in a one-minute news story, or even a readable newspaper article? They can't.

This loss of complexity isn't just the media's fault. Consider the type of articles you like to read, and the news program that you'll watch at 11:00 P.M. before going to bed. Do you want to plow through loads and loads of details, try to balance out the various probabilities and risks, consider the many possible alternative explanations of the data . . . and so on? No, you want a clear presentation of what's what. But *science rarely is able to give a clear "what's what."*

Scientists deal in probabilities. They won't say, "This product causes cancer," but rather, "There seems to be a relationship between this product and the growth of cancer cells in laboratory animals," or, "There is a 1 in 1,000 probability that exposure to this product will predispose an individual to cancer" — and that might require that the person has a host of other "predisposing conditions." Do you see how complicated it gets? As legal scholar Peter Huber wrote in *Galileo's Revenge: Junk Science in the Courtroom* (1991), "God is in the details, and nowhere is this more true than with the Creator's immutable laws of science."

Huber gives a real-life example of how the media scare us to death by ignoring the complexity of a health risk. The evening news anchorwoman says, with great concern in her expression, that women working at video display terminals (VDTs), such as computers, experience more miscarriages than women who don't work at these terminals.

Well, that's true. However, VDTs don't cause miscarriages. There isn't a direct cause-and-effect link. What has been proven to cause miscarriages is smoking, which increases the risk of miscarriage ten times. As Peter Huber points out, "Women who work outside the home smoke (or sit near a smoker) much more than others." So it isn't the VDT that causes miscarriages. Women who work at VDTs have a higher smoking rate, which increases miscarriages.

## WE *LIKE* HORROR MOVIES, VIOLENCE, MURDER, AND MAYHEM

The media aren't naive in choosing what to report. They know we like to be scared. Why do we read Stephen King novels? Why do we watch thriller movies that make it difficult for us to fall asleep at night? Why do we buy tabloids that scream, "Killer Bees on the Loose!"?

We like the adrenaline rush of fear. Therefore, in order to interest us enough to buy newspapers and think that "news" is essential, the media cover frightening and "sexy" risks.

Note how the media increase anxiety by highlighting the *risks* in headlines, as opposed to benefits. They don't report on the ways that technology makes our lives safer. No headline would say that five thousand commercial flights took place in the world yesterday, and none of the airplanes crashed — even though this headline describes the situation over 99 percent of the year.

## GIVE ME DRAMA, NOT NUMBERS

As the late Supreme Court justice Oliver Wendell Holmes put it, "Most people think dramatically, not quantitatively."

We hear about the abduction of a child on her way home from school and instantly worry about our child, even though tens of thousands of children walk home from school safely every day and the abduction took place in a distant city. The mere existence of the occurrence makes a stronger impression on us than the slim odds of that occurrence.

A comparison of news coverage of car crashes versus airplane crashes shows us how much the media favor the sensational story, even though statistics would work the other way. According to the *Los Angeles Times* (13 September 1994), our risk of dying in a car accident is about 1 in 6,000 — quite high, actually — while the risk of dying in a plane crash on a First World carrier is 1 in 4.4 million, or 1 in 11 million on a major carrier on a coast-to-coast flight. But the media devote a lot of attention to airplane crashes, and little or none to car crashes — because car crashes are so common. Therefore — *note the logical leap* — we worry about plane crashes.

## BESIDES—WHO REALLY WANTS TO READ *GOOD* NEWS?

Face it, good news is boring. Imagine a newspaper with these headlines: "People Enjoy Local Ice Cream Shop," with a subhead "Two Hundred Adults and Children Patronize Shop Each Day." Or, perhaps, "Double

Scoops More Popular than Single Scoops." Or, as another example, the "Lifestyle" section of the paper reports that most men and women rose from their beds the previous morning after a good night's sleep. The vast majority reached work safely after dropping their children off at school, where most of the kids are healthy and relatively happy. They all returned home at night, most of them safely. Very, very few died that night from clogged arteries or pesticide-provoked cancer. . . . Yawn.

Isn't this much more compelling? "Local Ice Cream Found to Cause Cancer," with a subheading of "Popular Flavors Contain Proven Carcinogen." Or "After-school Attacks on Children Rising."

Good news just doesn't get covered. Do you remember the now-famous pronouncements by the Center for Science in the Public Interest in 1993 and 1994 that ethnic foods — including Mexican, Chinese, and Italian dishes — are unhealthy? These sensational stories made front-page headlines around the country. Not much later, the Center for Science in the Public Interest released some good news. Their report on the "Top 10 Foods for Healthy Summer Fun" hardly got any press coverage at all. A newspaper in Dallas did cover it, but buried this story well within the paper.

Good news is just plain uninteresting. And yet "Studies have shown that people get more information about risk and hazard from the media than they do from their physicians or anyone else," says Walter Willett, professor of epidemiology and nutrition at the Harvard School of Public Health (reported by the *Los Angeles Times*, 12 September 1994). In fact, even government decision makers get a lot of their information from the media. Now *there's* something to be scared about.

## THE SQUEAKY WHEEL GETS THE PUBLIC SUPPORT

The media listen to whoever is loudest or more powerful. But loudness and power don't necessarily correlate with being right.

Take environmental groups. Whether they are right or not in their assertions, they clearly have media savvy. They have staged "media events" and protests, lobbied loudly, and published prolifically. They have "set the agenda," as media theorists say, by telling the public what's important. They don't just put their issues *in* the news; the issues *become* the news. That's more than half the battle toward swaying public opinion. And in these days when politicians listen more to the public pollster than to personal convictions of right or wrong, public opinion quickly becomes public policy, whether that opinion is correct or not.

## THE BIG MOUTH GETS THE MONEY

Scientists need research grants to survive. If a scientist says that her work has revealed dire possibilities for mankind unless more research is conducted, she is more likely to get funding for her future research. A doomsday scenario reported widely in the media is a surefire ticket to research support. Dr. Kenneth Olden, director of the National Institute of Environmental Health Sciences, admitted to the *Los Angeles Times* (13 September 1994) that "often scientists hype and build up their own findings [to get] . . . more funding."

Special interest groups and political activists have also learned to play the media in order to get more money. Media coverage is one reason why diseases such as AIDS and breast cancer get far more national research dollars than other diseases that kill more people. The *Los Angeles Times* (13 September 1994) compared breast cancer (forty-six thousand fatalities a year) and prostate cancer (thirty-eight thousand fatalities a year) in terms of media coverage and research dollars. In one year, breast cancer was mentioned 5,799 times in major newspaper and magazine articles. Prostate cancer had 1,742 mentions. Although breast cancer took only 22 percent more lives than prostate cancer, the media gave breast cancer 233 percent more coverage. What's the outcome of this media coverage? The National Cancer Institute put $213 million into breast cancer research, but only $51 million into prostate cancer research. That's a 418 percent difference in research dollars between diseases that are quite close in number of fatalities each year (*Los Angeles Times*, 13 September 1994).

## I'LL TAKE MY NEWS WITH A TEASPOON OF SKEPTICISM, PLEASE

Remember the movie *The Paper*, where the managing editor, played by Glenn Close, refused to stop the presses even though she knew that the cover story accused the wrong men of murder? She justified her decision by explaining that the paper could correct the mistake in the next edition on the following day.

That's callous and wrong, of course, but it illustrates a truth. The media often report news that is later proved inaccurate. They can't help it. Human beings can't see into the future. Philip Graham, the first publisher of the *Washington Post*, described a newspaper as "the inherent failings of the first rough draft of history."

Just how accurate are media stories on the dangers in our society? Two social scientists who specialize in risk, Dr. Eleanor Singer and Dr. Phyllis

Endreny, conducted a study of forty-two news stories, as described in their book *Reporting on Risk* (1993). They found that 76 percent had at least two errors!

By understanding the undisputed benefits as well as the *limitations* of television news, radio reports, magazines, and newspapers, we can become intelligent consumers of today's news — and maybe feel a little less scared.

# TECHNOLOGY: A DOUBLE-EDGED SWORD

How extraordinary! The richest, longest-lived, best protected, most resourceful civilization, with the highest degree of insight into its own technology, is on its way to becoming the most frightened.
—Aaron Wildavsky, political scientist, 1979, reported in the *Los Angeles Times*,
11 September 1994

If everything is as harmful as we're told, how come we're healthier and living longer . . . than ever before?
—Paul Portney, Vice President of Resources for the Future, a Washington think tank that specializes in environmental issues, reported in the *Los Angeles Times*,
12 September 1994

**M**odern technology is both the source of and solution to many of our fears today. Clearly it has benefited us. At the same time, technology raises new fears. Take a look at this brief list of ways that technology benefits us and the corresponding ways that each technology can scare us to death:

| BENEFITS | CORRESPONDING FEARS THAT TECHNOLOGY CAUSES OR NOW ALLOWS US TO SEE |
| --- | --- |
| Mammograms | Breast cancer |
| CAT scans | Other cancers |

| BENEFITS | CORRESPONDING FEARS THAT TECHNOLOGY CAUSES OR NOW ALLOWS US TO SEE |
|---|---|
| Antibiotics and dramatically increased longevity | Complacence among scientists; increased incidence of heart disease and cancer |
| Electricity | Risk of cancer from electromagnetic fields |
| Automobiles and personal mobility | Greenhouse effect, pollution, and more cancer |
| Computers | Yet more cancer from video displays |
| Electron microscopes | Pesticide residues (now visible) |
| Air travel | Airplane crashes and the rapid diffusion of infectious diseases |
| Air-conditioning and increased sanitation | Ozone depletion |
| Sophisticated chemical analysis | Toxicity of many everyday chemicals |
| Nuclear fission | Nuclear meltdown and catastrophe |
| Increase in skilled labor and economic prosperity | A widening gap between the rich and the poor; increased crime. |

As you can see, technology is a double-edged sword. It has made us healthier than ever before. We live longer. But it also creates risks and allows us to detect those risks more accurately than ever before.

Looking at technology in an overall cost-benefit analysis, the risks themselves have not increased. In fact, they've gone way, way down. We are safer, healthier, and wealthier than ever before. The industrialized world enjoys the highest standard of living in the history of our planet. But because technology allows us to see potential risks out there more than ever before, we've become more frightened.

## THE MICROSCOPE OF TECHNOLOGY: WE KNOW SO MUCH MORE

With modern technology, we can detect extremely tiny amounts of possibly harmful chemicals. Fifty, or even twenty, years ago we wouldn't have been able to notice them. Our parents ate fruit that carried pesticide residues, but no one knew it. While it's extremely beneficial that we can now detect the precise amount of pesticides that remain on food, and while it's good that we know the ill effects pesticides can bring, we have become terrified of any amount of pesticide as a result of our knowledge. That's not beneficial.

Medical advances have reduced or eliminated many of our historical risks. In the industrialized world, we no longer worry about polio, leprosy, or smallpox, for example. We have conquered many bacterial infections with antibiotics. If you have an ear infection, you go to the doctor, who takes a look inside and gives you antibiotics. Within a few days you're fine. You don't have to worry about a disease such as tonsillitis escalating into deadly scarlet fever — a threat your grandparents knew all too well.

Instead of being afraid of the legions of bacterial and viral illnesses that killed most of us a hundred years ago, we face a new menace: cancer. Why have cancer rates increased so much? With the eradication of traditional diseases and the improvements in our diets, we live much longer — so long, in fact, that we become old enough to contract diseases such as cancer. Legal scholar Peter Huber writes that "there is in fact a cancer epidemic, of sorts, caused (ironically) by the vaccines and antibiotics. Cancer is primarily a disease of old age; the most certain way to avoid it is to die young."

Technology has rid us of so many diseases that we are left with only a few. That fuels our fear of those few.

## TAKING TECHNOLOGY FOR GRANTED

The successes of modern technology have been so legion that we become horrified at the thought that technology might *not* save us. When a lethal new virus emerges in Africa and scientists don't know how to stop it, we are appalled and terrified. We take medical technology for granted and have come to think technology *should* save us. If it doesn't, we're angry. How dare there be risks in our society, given all those technological advances?

For example, when a baby dies at birth in a hospital (an uncommon occurrence today), rather than accepting the loss, some parents try to sue the doctors or the hospital. Peter Huber writes in *Galileo's Revenge: Junk Science in the Courtroom*, "Modern medical science compounds the problem by reason of its very successes: obstetricians have become so skilled at saving babies that their failures are all the harder to accept." We have come to believe that we and our loved ones should be safe at all times.


## THE LUXURY OF WORRY

Do people in Somalia worry about traces of Alar or other pesticides on food? Do villagers in rural India lose sleep over the possibility of asbestos fibers in the air? Would a small village in Borneo be concerned about the possible electromagnetic fields radiating from the electrical wire recently brought to town, or happy that electricity finally came, bringing with it light and refrigeration, and with *them* improved sanitation and a better overall quality of life? Are inhabitants of the desert of northern Africa anxious about trace chemicals in their water supply?

Hardly. In the industrialized world we have the luxury of worrying about protection from trace elements, invisible radiation fields, minuscule risks from building materials, and so forth. It can be useful to put our fears in perspective. While it's worthwhile to continue examining the safety of our society (that's in part what led us to our current comfort), it can be enlightening to see how privileged we are. Maybe the "scares" we face aren't so bad after all.


## THIS "NEWFANGLED THING" CAN'T POSSIBLY BE ANY GOOD . . .

Does this sound like your crotchety grandfather's complaints about some new piece of technology? Why would he be so negative about anything new? Could it be because he's afraid? The innovative piece of new technology might be beyond his current comprehension. In short, it's new. Whatever's new is always a bit scary — whether it's a new job, a new relationship, or a new city.

Most of us have a bit of the crotchety old man in us. People tend to be nervous about any new technology. Undoubtedly the caveman who invented the wheel was warned by a neighbor that his invention would bring an end to civilization, or at least would crush someone's feet if the wheels went out of control. Thomas Edison was warned against the dangers of developing electricity for widespread use.

Yes, we could electrocute ourselves by sticking our finger into a live socket. But electricity has saved countless lives. Aren't we much better off with electricity than without? Isn't it better to pursue new technologies intelligently, measuring risks and benefits, and not overreact to those risks before examining the benefits? The same might be said of nuclear power, X-ray technology, and genetic engineering of food.

Technology exists to serve human beings. With awareness of the strengths, limitations, and social dynamics of technology, we can use it to help us (its original purpose), not scare us.

# HUMAN PSYCHOLOGY IN THE MODERN AGE

The risks that kill people and the risks that scare people are different.
—Peter Sandman, risk communications consultant, quoted in the *Los Angeles Times*, 11 September 1994

**H**uman psychology is a strange phenomenon. We're willing to go bungee jumping off a cliff, but we're furious at a possible trace of pesticide on an apple in the grocery store. We fear flying on airplanes, but we speed on the Interstate and sometimes don't wear our seat belts. We become horrified when we hear that fettuccine Alfredo is "a heart attack on a plate" (as quoted from the *Los Angeles Times*, 11 September 1994) in fat content, but we willingly eat fluorescent orange barbecue-flavored potato chips fried in coconut oil.

We're afraid to watch the evening news when we're alone in our house, so we keep a handgun at home — in spite of the well-documented increase in deadly violence in homes where a handgun is kept for protection. We sue the local power company over the much-debated electromagnetic fields supposedly radiating from high-frequency lines, and then race our bicycle down a hill without wearing a helmet.

The U.S. Department of Transportation estimates that the increased preference for smaller cars leads to thirteen hundred deaths annually. Of course, we all know that smaller cars are more dangerous, but we trade off safety for greater fuel efficiency. Those little convertibles and sports cars have great style, too. We each believe that we wouldn't be hurt seriously in an accident thanks to our cute small car. Those things happen to someone else.

In her book *Risk Acceptability According to the Social Sciences* (1985), anthropologist Mary Douglas put it bluntly: "Put to the test formally humans do not seem to be good at rational thinking."

Researchers on risk have identified dozens of odd bits of human behavior that illustrate how we interpret fears. For example:

- We tend to overestimate the dangers of rare events while dismissing the dangers of more-common events. For instance, we fear flying in airplanes but not driving, which is actually far more dangerous. The FDA reported that ironically the risks associated with a high-fat, low-fiber diet are more acceptable in the public's mind than the risk posed by Alar (Phyllis M. Endreny, *Reporting on Risk: How the Mass Media Portrays Accidents, Disease and Other Hazards.* New York, Russell Sage Foundation, 1993).

- We often assume that when we can control a situation, we're more likely to be safe. However, the high number of fatalities in automobile accidents illustrates that just because we're behind the wheel, it doesn't mean we're safe.

- We think that when a situation is familiar, there's nothing to fear. But an experienced rock climber's single deadly slip proves that familiarity doesn't necessarily mean safety. And statistics continue to show that most accidents happen in or near the familiar surroundings of our own home.

- We're much less likely to fear the possibility of natural disasters — earthquakes, floods, tornadoes, hurricanes, fires — than man-made disasters. We also feel less angry about natural disasters. If we lose a limb from a surgeon's ineptness or a dangerous product, we file expensive lawsuits. On the other hand, if we lose a limb by being crushed in a building during an earthquake, we move on with our lives much more easily.

- We're more worried by dramatic but infrequent events, such as sudden outbreaks of rare viruses, than by more "boring" risks, like being killed by slipping in the bathtub.

Why do we behave so strangely? Aren't we logical at all?

Risk consultant Peter Sandman believes that people's fears about various potential risks in society reflect "outrage" more than the actual degree of hazard. People believe that life can and should be risk-free. We want life, liberty, and the pursuit of happiness. More than "want," we believe that these are our *rights*.

Our society has become so safe and successful that we believe most dangers should be eliminated by now. For example, we're so horrified at the thought of toxic waste left at dumping grounds that we spend a billion dollars cleaning up the last 1 percent when we could have cleaned up 90 percent for only $10 million (*Los Angeles Times*, 12 September 1994). Absolute zero risk is impossible, but we are determined to come as close to that as time, money, and technology will permit.

Another human tendency is to prefer a clear right and wrong. We want answers, not philosophical or scientific uncertainty. Consultant Peter Sandman tells how former senator Edmund Muskie would become frustrated with the necessary qualifications and uncertainties in science. When scientists qualified their statements with the phrase "on the other hand," Muskie allegedly retorted, "Find me an expert with one hand."

A related explanation for why we are scaring ourselves to death is that people tend to make quick leaps to conclusions. We're a culture of fast food, ATM machines, direct deposit, faxes, and e-mail. We work fast, move fast, and want absolute answers fast. Unfortunately, science moves at a painstakingly slow pace. It can take years for a study to arrive at reliable conclusions, and even more time for other scientists to replicate the study to see if the conclusions hold. Possible intervening variables are also examined. . . . Decades sometimes pass before valid conclusions can be drawn. The scientific process is meticulous, but we don't want to wait.

Humans also like to search for the good guy and the bad guy in every situation. We want to find someone to blame for our misfortunes. By externalizing risks — in other words, making something outside ourselves responsible — we set ourselves up for fear, but also allow ourselves to blame someone else when things go wrong.

In another book, *Risk and Blame* (1992), Mary Douglas describes the "blaming system" of today as "almost ready to treat every death as chargeable to someone's account, every accident as caused by someone's criminal negligence, every sickness a threatened prosecution. Whose fault? is the first question. Then, what action? Which means, what damages? what compensation? what restitution?"

Legal scholar Peter Huber points out in *Galileo's Revenge* that "blaming something or other, no matter how far off base scientifically, brings meaning to otherwise senseless suffering, and the meaning seems to supply some measure of comfort. Still more comfort may be at hand when the returns . . . are paid in cash."

Cynical? Perhaps. But we've become cynical, disbelieving the government's promise to protect us. That's another reason we're scared to death.

After Watergate and Vietnam, and with all the political scandals these days, we no longer believe that government can take care of things. Corporations are even worse, lying through their teeth about the efficacy and "safety" of their products. Whom do we believe? By default, we gather most of our information from the media.

The media, however, have bombarded us with so much that we begin to feel helpless, unable to sort through all the conflicting reports. We receive so much information in this "information age" that a new term has been coined: *information overload*. When people are overloaded, they tend to give up, when, in fact, there are steps we can take to protect ourselves from the real risks.

We've become so hypersensitive to dangers that it seems impossible to avoid calamity. In *Risk and Blame*, Mary Douglas describes how "protecting against one category of risk exposes one to another. For example, preventing risks of fire or riot requires open access to the premises; but risks of stolen information call for restricted access: you can have one, or the other, but not both." If you protect your house by putting bars on all the windows, you could die in a fire from smoke inhalation while trying to push open the bars. If you avoid eating vegetables out of fear of pesticides, you lose the excellent health benefits of vegetables, including protection against cancer — the very thing you were trying to achieve by avoiding pesticides! If you fear leaving the house at night because of crime, you can begin to feel lonely and depressed — emotional states that carry high prices for our health.

Is there no way to assess the dangers of modern life calmly and clearly? How can we avoid the two extremes of ignoring the real risks that exist, and scaring ourselves to death? By becoming aware of our quirky human psychology in this age of media frenzy and sophisticated technology, we can begin to put our fears in perspective.

Think about your relationship to fear. What do you gain, and lose, by holding certain fears? Where are your fears founded, and where not? What impact does fear have on your life? Are you scaring yourself to death? If so, can you arrive at an intelligent, comfortable approach to enjoying *life* more? The following information will help you get there.

# TO YOUR
# HEALTH!

# HEALTHY, WEALTHY, AND WISE (?)

Tylenol poisonings. AIDS. Rare killer viruses with no cures. Hamburgers that kill children and old people. Beef that makes you mad. Salmonella-contaminated chicken in the local grocery store. Pesticides on fruits and vegetables. Toxic shellfish. Milk pumped up with bovine growth hormones. Mexican food, Italian food, Chinese food, movie theater popcorn. According to media stories over the past few years, all of these are "harmful to your health"!

To add to the confusion, sometimes one piece of health news is followed within weeks by another that directly contradicts the first.

- In February 1995, the Centers for Disease Control told us that any kind of exercise improved life expectancy, even sporadic modest exercise. Then, two months later, a Harvard University study announced that only people who exercised strenuously and regularly enjoyed longer lives.
- A Danish study, published in the 6 May 1995 issue of the *British Medical Journal,* encourages the drinking of wine. According to the ten-year study, people who drink three to five glasses of wine a day live longer. However, other studies point out that the benefits of alcohol might not outweigh the risks.
- One study finds that eating fish doesn't prevent heart disease, as it is widely believed to do. Another study reports that reducing dietary fat to 30 percent of calorie intake doesn't help reduce the risk of heart disease — in spite of dozens of news stories to the contrary.

It's difficult to know what to embrace and what to fear. Questions cloud our attempts to apply the results of scientific research to our lives. We learn that food irradiation can kill potentially harmful bacteria, such as *E. coli* in beef and pork, and salmonella in chicken. But does irradiation carry unforeseen cancer risks?

Another example is caffeine. Eighty percent of Americans consume caffeine daily. However, a Johns Hopkins University report published in the *Journal of the American Medical Association* in October 1994 found that caffeine causes birth defects and is an addictive drug with classical psychoactive dependence. Other studies tell us that caffeine magnifies the risk of heart attacks and the effects of stress. Conversely, different researchers and food professionals assert that caffeine can *protect* against colon and rectal cancer, increase alertness and productivity, reduce suicidal tendencies, and increase sexual activity in the elderly. So what do we do, have that second cup of coffee or not?

And what is the difference between saturated fat, unsaturated fat, and polyunsaturated fat? Does fluoride help our teeth, or hurt our kidneys?

Help! We're continually bombarded with advice on health issues. A recent *New York Times* headline (10 May 1995) read, "Amid Inconclusive Health Studies, Some Experts Advise Less Advice"!

The overabundance of health advice can, itself, be harmful to our health. Dr. Donald Louria, chairman of preventive medicine and community health at the New Jersey Medical School in Newark, told the *New York Times* (10 May 1995) that "the danger of [overselling health advice to the public] is that they will not believe the stuff we have that's documented." In other words, the bona fide, scientifically sound health advice gets lost in the crowd. Another physician, Dr. Walter Willett of the Harvard School of Public Health, worries about the "lack of distinction between wishful thinking and solid facts in health advice. When a new study contradicts conventional wisdom, people throw up their hands and decide not to believe anything scientists say" (*New York Times*, 10 May 1995).

The good news is that our health has never been better in the history of mankind! According to the National Center for Health Statistics, as recently as 1890 the average life expectancy for Americans was just over 31 years old. By 1930, the average life lasted just under 60 years — almost doubling in only forty years. By 1990, the average life expectancy had reached 75.4, the highest in history. Infant deaths have dropped by half over the past twenty years, to just over 9 babies in every 100,000 born today (*Los Angeles Times*, 11 September 1994).

In addition, the death rate from heart disease (the No. 1 killer) has dropped

27 percent since 1970. Deaths from stroke (the No. 3 killer) are down 44 percent. Smallpox is gone, and polio is almost gone. We can cure leprosy. Cancer deaths (the No. 2 killer) have increased, but this rise is mostly due to smoking and to the fact that we're living longer; other diseases don't get us first.

Nevertheless, in spite of this overwhelmingly good news, 78 percent of Americans still think that they face more risk than their parents did twenty years ago, according to researchers Marsh and McLennan in the *Los Angeles Times* (11 September 1994). Only 6 percent think that we face less risk. Why is this? It seems that we're scaring ourselves to death. The following information can help us sort through some of the many "scare stories" and the conflicting advice about our health.

# BREAST CANCER SCARE

*U*.S. News and World Report describes "a breast-cancer epidemic": "Every three minutes, a woman is diagnosed, and every 11 minutes, a woman dies from the disease. It strikes one in eight women and kills 46,000 a year" (23 November 1992).

The National Breast Cancer Coalition sends a fundraising letter to millions of Americans. The letter reads, "We are at *war*. And our enemy is breast cancer. It attacks women brutally and indiscriminately. It has reached *epidemic proportions* in America. . . . And if you think you're safe because breast cancer doesn't run in your family, think again. Three-quarters of new cases are diagnosed in women who have *no family history* of the disease."

The concerns about breast cancer being reported in the media are important. This dreaded disease is deadly, disfiguring, and physically and emotionally painful even if "cured." It's true that breast cancer is on the rise. At the same time, women can't walk around in terror of breast cancer. In fact, many studies have shown that anxiety predisposes people to diseases such as heart disease and even cancer.

Let's try to sort through the rhetoric on breast cancer to identify the real risks and arrive at an intelligent approach for women to prevent the disease.

*Outlook* (6 May 1995) reports on how the *Women's Health Letter* breaks down that famous "one in eight women" statistic. Those 1-in-8 odds refer only to women who live to be ninety-five. Three-quarters of diagnosed breast cancers occur in women over fifty. Breast cancer is *primarily* a disease of elderly women. Thanks to medical advances, we have more elderly people alive today in our society than ever before in history. If we have more cases of breast cancer, it's because we have more older women. *That's* the "epidemic."

It's true that there are more cases of breast cancer in young women than there were sixty years ago, because there are more younger women today, especially the baby boomers. Our population has increased. The *number* of cases has grown, but the *rate* of cases — the *percentage* of people in that group who get breast cancer — has not changed. The actual risk itself hasn't increased.

The *Women's Health Letter* (6 May 1995) stated that the 1-in-8 statistic doesn't describe a woman's immediate risk. Rather, women have different risks at different ages, with the risk increasing as a woman ages. Specifically, according to a chart developed by the National Cancer Institute, "A 20-year-old woman has a 1-in-2,500 chance of developing breast cancer. At age 30, it's 1 in 233. At age 40, it's 1 in 63. At age 50, it's 1 in 41. At age 60, it's 1 in 28. At age 70, it's 1 in 24. At age 80, it's 1 in 16. And at age 95, it's 1 in 8."

Another reason why we might seem to be having a breast cancer epidemic is related to the sophistication of our medical technology. A specialist in breast cancer at the University of Southern California, Dr. Malcolm Pike, told the *Los Angeles Times* (13 September 1994) that "there's been an enormous increase in screening, in early detection, an enormous increase in the number of mammographic machines around." Dr. Pike believes that most of the increase in breast cancer cases is due to the increase in detection. We can't name something and turn it into a statistic if we don't know it's there. Sixty years ago, if a woman died of breast cancer, we might not have known what caused her death. Now we know.

This same medical technology that increases the statistics on *cases* of breast cancer also decreases the statistics on *deaths* from breast cancer. The National Cancer Institute (*Los Angeles Times*, 11 January 1995) reports that breast cancer deaths dropped 6 percent from 1989 to 1992 (only three years) because more women were screened and treated. Women whose breast cancer is detected early have up to a 93 percent chance of survival.

One of the problems in coping with the fear of breast cancer has been mixed messages from the experts. Just as a woman is about to rush out to get a mammogram to assure herself that she doesn't have breast cancer, she hears that mammograms might increase the risk of cancer because of the radiation in the X ray. In fact, the National Cancer Institute argues *against* women under fifty having mammograms. The woman rushes back home, only to read in the newspaper the next day that the American Medical Association and the American Cancer Society say that women in their forties *should* have mammograms.

Why so much media attention and so many mixed messages about breast cancer? Consider who is reporting the news. Four out of 10 newsroom workers are women, and many women feel (perhaps correctly) that women's health issues haven't received a fair shake from the media and thus from government funding. Breast cancer has become more than a health issue that reflects the actual incidence of the disease. It is a political issue. For that reason it gets more coverage than it otherwise would.

Breast cancer is also what journalists call a "sexy" issue — one that grabs attention. For example, a movie about a woman fighting breast cancer would receive more attention from the general public than a movie about a woman fighting heart problems, even though heart disease kills more women each year than breast cancer. Breasts are sexual; they have deep reproductive significance; they are central to a woman's own sense of her attractiveness; they flounce through men's fantasies. In American culture (unlike many others) women cover their breasts, implicitly making them even more special, not to be revealed to just anyone. Breasts *are* special to us; breast cancer, therefore, is also special (and especially frightening).

How about the allegation from environmentalists that pesticides have contributed to the so-called breast cancer epidemic? Research answers with a resounding no. The largest study ever on breast cancer was conducted by the Mayo Clinic in 1994. This study found no evidence that pesticides in our food cause breast cancer. Still, the proposition that pesticides cause breast cancer is another of the many scares put forth by environmentalists.

In fact, we might argue that indirectly, at least, pesticides help *prevent* breast cancer. Pesticides help farmers produce low-cost and plentiful fruits and vegetables. Many studies have shown that eating vegetables and fruit protects people from cancer. The *Los Angeles Times* (19 January 1995) reported on a recent Greek study that found that eating vegetables reduced a woman's risk of breast cancer by 12 percent. Fruits help prevent breast cancer by 8 percent. If a woman avoids fruits and vegetables because of the media's reports linking pesticides and cancer, she may be truly "scaring herself to death."

Let's get back to the quandary faced by the forty-year-old woman considering a mammogram. *Should* women under fifty have regular mammograms? Breast cancer might not be an epidemic, but it's still a risk, right? That's true — a risk that varies in seriousness for different women. If a younger woman has a family history (i.e., "high risk") of breast cancer, she should have mammograms. If she doesn't have this history and is under fifty, experts argue that she can probably go either way, depending on how "safe" she wants to feel and how much money she wants to spend. Mammograms cost money. Generally speaking, mammograms for low-risk women under forty don't make economic sense because mammography for women in this age group has not been shown to save any lives, according to a recent study by RAND, the think tank based in Santa Monica, California. Also, the composition of younger women's breasts makes it harder to see tiny tumors.

Women should *not* avoid mammograms because of fear of the radiation in X rays. The risk of the X ray pales in comparison to the benefit of the mammogram, even for women under forty. So if the X ray is the only thing coming between you and a mammogram that you should have, you're *hurting* not helping yourself.

For young women who are afraid to do breast self-examinations in the shower and in front of the mirror, take courage: you're very unlikely to find a tumor. But you *will* become more familiar with your breasts so that you won't panic one morning when you snap on your bra and think you feel a little knot that, in reality, has been there all the time. You'll also know what your breasts are like so that as you age, entering into higher risk groups, you can (quite literally) save yourself from invasive breast cancer.

# AMPLE ENDOWMENT: THE PUMPED-UP HYSTERIA
## OVER BREAST IMPLANTS

The largest product-liability settlement in American history — $4.25 billion — was reached in September 1994. Over ninety thousand women have filed claims to receive compensation awards ranging from $105,000 to $1.4 million, depending on their medical condition and their age when their symptoms first appeared. While the final disposition of this case is still uncertain — plaintiffs, claims administrators, and lawyers are still haggling over many parts of it — it is clear at this point that the companies involved in making breast implants will be shelling out at least the $4.25 billion already agreed to in the settlement.

Why are these women being awarded such ample endowments? Because, they claim, their health has been placed at severe risk by the breast implants they received. They claim that their implants cause cancer, rheumatoid arthritis, short-term memory disorders, lupus, other immune disorders, and fevers, aches, and chills. They assert that the main manufacturer of breast implants, Dow Corning, hid scientific evidence for twenty years that silicone, the most important ingredient in implants, suppresses the immune system.

It would seem that a settlement of $4.25 billion implies an admission of guilt by Dow Corning. But this isn't the case. Dow Corning (and other manufacturers of breast implants and their components) agreed to the settlement to avoid the legal costs of individual lawsuits, but they do not admit that breast implants cause harm. On the contrary. The companies insist that breast implants don't cause cancer, immune system disorders, or any of the other diseases claimed by the women.

The implant manufacturers aren't simply trying to deny guilt. There is strong medical evidence that implants don't cause the symptoms claimed by the women. This should come as good news to the two million women who have implants, and who have been unnecessarily terrified by the hype against implants.

Doctors have also contributed to the hype. Many of them have their own agendas behind either banning or promoting implants. For example, The *Los Angeles Times* (9 September 1994) ran an op-ed piece by Dr. Samuel Epstein, a public health professor at the University of Illinois at Chicago and chairman of the Cancer Prevention Coalition. Dr. Epstein claims that breast implants, particularly polyurethane-wrapped implants, are horribly dangerous and that Dow Corning is a first-class villain. As Dr. Epstein put it, "Polyurethane-wrapped implants are . . . carcinogenic sponges." That's a highly politicized way of discussing risks, even if it were true.

To the *Los Angeles Times'* (30 September 1994) credit, a couple of weeks later they printed a reply from Dr. Dennis Deapen, a researcher from the University of Southern California. Dr. Deapen insisted that Dr. Epstein blatantly ignored "the strong and consistent evidence that breast implants do not cause cancer in humans." Dr. Deapen pointed out that no breast cancers have been reported among the tens of thousands of women who have received polyurethane-covered implants — supposedly the most carcinogenic kind of implant. In fact, he says that breast implant patients in general develop "significantly fewer breast cancers than expected." Moreover, despite the FDA's decision to ban implants in 1992, an FDA panel of experts concluded that the risk of implants was negligible and recommended that implants remain available to women.

It's important to recognize that the FDA is currently extremely conservative and eager to ban anything that poses *any* potential risk at all. The FDA has also become so ultraconservative about approving anything without extensive testing that it's almost impossible to bring new products to market. In fact, Republicans in Congress, including House Speaker Newt Gingrich, want to do away with the FDA because (as they claim) the FDA prevents useful devices from being made available to the public. Therefore, just because the FDA bans something, such as breast implants, that doesn't mean the product is necessarily dangerous. It simply means that the FDA is being careful.

More and more evidence shows that the FDA might have overreacted. In 1994, researchers at Massachusetts General Hospital conducted a preliminary study of 32 women (26 with breast implants) that found that silicone seeping into the body from implants might actually help *combat* breast cancer. A second study of 5 women with implants found that the plasma from 3 of the women who had their implants for over a decade was able to kill the cancer cells. This study, and others like it, are leading scientists to consider how silicone might be used to help fight cancer in general (*Los Angeles Times*, 10 August 1994).

Researchers at Harvard University recently published the results of the largest study ever on the relationship between breast implants and immune disorders such as those claimed by the plaintiffs in the Dow Corning lawsuit. While an initial look at the numbers might be shocking (a 24 percent increase in the risk of disease), these statistics need a closer scrutiny. Although 24 percent increase seems an astoundingly high number, one must be aware that in the general population, the risk of these diseases is extremely low, only .114 percent. This means that in women with breast implants the increased incidence of these diseases is only 1 case per 3,000 (*Wall Street Journal*, 28 February 1996).

Furthermore, the Mayo Clinic conducted another large study of women with breast implants. This study found absolutely no evidence that implants cause any of the diseases claimed by the women. (Several other large studies also showed no association between implants and the diseases.) The Mayo Clinic researchers claim that the diseases contracted by the women who won the $4.25 billion could be completely unrelated to their implants. Indeed, until the Mayo Clinic study, no one had ever conducted a scientific comparison of the general health of women with implants versus women without implants (*Los Angeles Times*, 16 June 1994)!

Then why did Dow Corning and the other manufacturers agree to pay women with breast implants all this money? Do these women have a case?

Their case rests on the fact that Dow Corning didn't reveal a research study, conducted at their laboratories in 1975, that showed a relationship between silicone and cancer. This study matters, the women say, because silicone breast implants sometimes leak or rupture. Silicone can then travel through the body and cause all sorts of health problems, including cancer.

It's true that Dow Corning didn't exactly highlight this study when the FDA conducted an earlier examination of breast implants in 1987. It did mention the study, but only briefly, explaining that it didn't pertain to breast implants.

A look at the study itself will show why Dow Corning said that it wasn't relevant. In 1975, Dow Corning conducted a study of the effects of silicone injected into mice. The purpose of the study was to see if silicone could be used as a medicine. The mice in the study developed malignant tumors. This seems to establish a strong connection between leaking implants and cancer, doesn't it?

Not necessarily. The mice received D4, a purified form of silicone found in very tiny amounts in the implants. By itself, D4 didn't hurt the mice at all. Only when D4 was combined with another chemical, which is not included in implants, did it harm the mice. Even then, the harm was only temporary. Still, an independent evaluation of the study concluded that high levels of D4 were toxic, and this was sufficient to provide a basis for the lawsuit.

The final argument used by the women is that the carcinogenic effects of implants might require thirty years or more to show up, like the effects of asbestos and dioxin. That may be the case; we just don't know yet. However, hundreds of thousands of women have received breast implants in the last thirty years. Thus far, there is no direct proof that breast implants cause any disease.

Who really benefits in the breast implant battle? Not the women, even though those who truly are ill will receive the largest amounts of money, whether or not their illnesses were caused by the implants. Money can never compensate for what they've suffered.

Rather, it's the lawyers who are going to become truly "amply endowed." Right after the settlement was approved, the big topic of discussion became how much of that money the lawyers would get. The women are trying to limit it to $1 billion of the $4.25 billion. Overall, the breast implant litigation and settlement took two years to resolve, and it may take another year for the claims administrator to evaluate the validity of all the claims. A billion dollars for a few years' work isn't bad.

# AN APPLE A DAY . . .

. . . causes cancer?

According to a now-famous *60 Minutes* broadcast in February 1989, the "most potent cancer-causing agent in our food supply is a substance sprayed on apples. . . ." *60 Minutes* warned that this substance — Alar — was especially dangerous to children.

Hearing those words, mothers across the country snatched the apples out of their kids' lunch boxes. Grocery stores around the nation pulled apples off the shelves. Bachelors threw cans of apple juice concentrate out of their freezers. School boards banned apples from their school lunch programs. Health-conscious organic types, who really did eat an apple a day, felt suddenly nauseated at the thought of what they'd done.

What *60 Minutes* didn't say was that, although apple growers had in fact already moved away from using Alar, it had once been used to keep apples longer on the tree and make them look prettier. The program also didn't say that scientists were uncertain about any health hazards caused by Alar, and that scientific studies contradicted each other. But that didn't stop the media machine from revving into high gear.

The Alar scare is a classic case of how the media can create mass hysteria and cause far more damage than the alleged culprit ever could.

Why was the Alar story such a media gold mine? It had two of the media's favorite attention-grabber words — *children* and *cancer*. These were coupled with that most American of concepts, the apple — part of apple pie, Johnny Appleseed, Washington and Vermont autumns, pork chops and applesauce.

Who actually suffered most as a result of the Alar scare? To begin with, we did. Most of us became unnecessarily scared of a healthy, nutritious food.

Second, we allowed the media to tell us what was dangerous, rather than science. *That's* more dangerous as a precedent than any Alar-sprayed apple. And finally, the apple industry lost more than $100 million and dumped billions of apples. Some smaller apple growers were even forced out of business.

It's more than just a shame that all this had to happen, especially because the evidence against Alar wasn't absolutely sound. The U.S. Environmental Protection Agency had been investigating Alar, but the evidence was so incomplete that they had decided there was no rush to take any action.

Even the U.S. surgeon general, C. Everett Koop, whom the public viewed with esteem and trusted as the protector of the public health, wasn't worried about Alar. Dr. Koop explained in 1992 why he didn't jump onto the Alar-scare bandwagon: "If Alar ever posed a health hazard, I would have said so then and would say so now. When used in the regulated, approved manner, as Alar was before it was withdrawn in 1989, Alar-treated apple products posed no hazards to the health of children or adults."

According to biochemist Bruce Ames of the *FDA Consumer* (June 1990), the risk of cancer from Alar is about the same as from tap water (which contains chloroform) — and, in fact, is about thirty times lower than the risk from peanut butter (which contains aflatoxin, a natural carcinogen).

So there we have it. As one of the directors at the National Cancer Institute, Dr. Richard Adamson, put it, the risk of eating an apple sprayed with Alar was "certainly less than the risk of eating a well-done hamburger."

In 1989, during the Alar scare, its manufacturer pulled it off the market. But it wasn't until 1992 — three years later — that the EPA officially banned Alar (a bit of a moot point, wasn't it?). The EPA proclaimed that Alar "posed an unreasonable risk of cancer to the public." Realistically, despite the opinions of experts such as the surgeon general, the EPA *had* to condemn Alar — or look foolish, given the public uproar that had occurred. Worse yet, the EPA would look like a puppet of pesticide companies, which would play right into the hands of environmental groups.

Ultimately, what really happened in the Alar wars is that one special interest group "won": the environmentalists. They played on the media's favorite buzzwords (*children* and *cancer*), manipulated the EPA into taking a public stance against Alar, and struck the fear of pesticides into our hearts. The Alar scare made us more aware of the possible dangers of pesticides than ever before. That's just what the environmentalists wanted. They dangled bait — an Alar-sprayed apple — in front of the media, and the media bit.

In the end, the advice still holds true: "An apple a day keeps the doctors away." Apples are an excellent source of fiber and many vitamins. The benefits of eating apples far, far outweigh any possible risk you might incur. So pack those apples in kids' school lunches, bring an apple to work, bake apple pies, drink apple juice, and enjoy.

# SOUR GRAPES

**H**ow many cyanide-laced grapes does it take to kill someone? A bunch? Ten? How about if the amount of cyanide isn't even close to lethal? How many grapes does it take then?

In 1989, two grapes — yes, two — from Chile were found to contain non-lethal amounts of cyanide. As a result, the U.S. Food and Drug Administration pulled all fruit from Chile off supermarket shelves and stopped all imports. The cost to the U.S. economy was at least $20 million, according to the *New Republic* (1 May 1989). That's $10 million per grape — and these two grapes weren't going to hurt anyone even if they were plucked and eaten.

Why did the government overreact so much? Well, imagine the accusations that would be flung at government officials if they knowingly let those two grapes show up in a store: "The U.S. government doesn't care about the public's health." The president and his cabinet officials might be blamed for being "unresponsive to public needs." Various members of Congress would make soapbox speeches about the imperative to protect the public good. . . .

All over two little grapes.

Maybe some judicious testing of samples of the fruit at different locations around the country would have been a more appropriate approach for the FDA to take.

But consumers also reacted. Grapes sales were down for months. What could happen to two grapes could happen to any grape, right? Even out of *millions* of grapes. Why did we overreact when we heard that two grapes contained trace amounts of cyanide?

We fear that the two-grapes-out-of-a-million could end up on our plate. And what if there are more than two? How do we know there aren't others? What if there's a conspiracy by Chilean extremists to kill us? Maybe we also should give up Chilean black beans. How about Chilean sea bass? And orange juice, too; some of the oranges in that concentrate in your freezer come from South America. . . .

Whoa! Look at it this way. You don't quit your job and stay home for the rest of your life even though people are killed on their way to work in car accidents *every day*. You don't stop eating meat because someone was once poisoned by it — or avoid wheat because once there was a bug in the flour — or fruit because you once bought a peach that had a worm. Of course not. Life *is* risk. And when the risk is 1 grape in 1 million, the odds aren't bad.

On a larger scale, think about the possible repercussions of our overreactions. Aren't we giving a little too much power to terrorists and maniacs? If one person tampers with Tylenol and we pull Tylenol off the shelves, we are being careful with the public's health, but we're also giving tremendous power to that terrorist. And all the people who need Tylenol because they can't take aspirin are out of luck.

It's true that many things can kill us. Every object and experience harbors hidden danger. Will that danger step out of the shadows and strike *you*? Will the two grapes in a million end up on *your* plate? Maybe. Does that mean that you'll never eat another grape for fear of cyanide, or never go outside for fear of murder, or never touch another person for fear of contracting a rare infectious disease? We hope not. Helen Keller put it best: "Life is either a daring adventure, or it is nothing."

# FEAR OF FAT

**O**ne of the worst fears that individuals have in our modern society is FAT. We dread becoming fat. Diet books sell by the millions of copies as the public eagerly reads how to eat and cook in low-fat ways. Thousands of young women become anorexic each year because they fear becoming fat. People pay hundreds of dollars to visit "fat farms," where they can exercise strenuously, eat low-fat or no-fat foods, receive nutritional advice, and (hopefully) lose a few pounds. New Year's resolutions typically involve a pledge to lose weight. Thousands of television programs, magazine articles, and newspaper stories tell us how to avoid the "f" word: FAT.

"Fear of fat" truly illustrates how we're scaring ourselves to death — literally, in the case of anorexic and bulimic young women. But Americans' fear of fat isn't shared around the world. In other countries, particularly in the Third World, chubbiness is seen as a sign of wealth (indicating the ability to grow or purchase food). Only in countries of wealth and abundance is fat feared.

How bad is fat *really?*

Media reports make fat sound really, really bad. Fear of fat hogged the headlines when the Center for Science in the Public Interest (CSPI) slammed Chinese, Italian, and Mexican food for its high fat content. Fettuccine Alfredo was called "A HEART ATTACK ON A PLATE" (Center for Science in the Public Interest as quoted in the *Los Angeles Times*, 11 September 1994). The CSPI equated a dinner-size serving of fettucine Alfredo, at 97 grams of fat, with eating a full stick of butter. Two chile rellenos with beans and rice are only a little less bad — about a quarter-pound stick of butter, or 92 grams of fat. Chimichanga: 86 grams. Kung pao chicken: 76 grams, or the equivalent of four McDonald's Quarter Pounders.

Worst of all was the CSPI's popcorn study. A medium tub of buttered pop-corn at movie theaters, they reported, has "more fat than a bacon-and-egg breakfast, a Big Mac-with-fries and a steak dinner with all the trimmings . . . combined." As columnist and humorist Dave Barry wrote, "You got the im-pression from the wildly excited press coverage that after a movie ends the ushers have to use forklifts to clear the bloated corpses out of the theater."

It's true that excessive fat intake is linked to cancer and heart disease. The non-fat and low-fat food trend is positive in that it does help to improve our health. The media blitzes by the Center for Science in the Public Interest have led movie theaters to switch from saturated-fat coconut oil to health-ier alternatives in making popcorn. Supermarkets have introduced health foods. McDonald's and other fast-food chains now present lower-fat alter-natives, including low-fat burgers and fat-free muffins.

However, this dietary craze against fat can go too far. We *need* fat. Women need body fat in order to have children, and our skin needs body fat to re-tain elasticity. There are other benefits to fat as well. How have we come to see fat as an enemy to be vanquished at all costs?

The no-fat/low-fat trend has the same impetus as other food trends throughout history: in the human desire to figure out ways to live longer, to be healthier, and to meet with social approval. It can be amusing to look at dietary advice of the past to see how *wrong* such advice later proved to be. For example, it was once believed that salt and other condiments cause in-sanity. Cooked vegetables were "against God's law." Food gurus of the past once believed that consumption of fourteen pounds of strawberries and grapes a day lowers blood pressure. Slow, methodical chewing lowers blood pressure. Grape Nuts cures malaria. Fasting and then eating as many grapes as possible will cure cancer. Eating starches with anything else (especially protein with carbohydrates) could lead to a "digestive explosion." Honey and meat served rare can prevent aging, loss of sexual potency, and premature death. Vitamin C cures back pain and viruses. Drinking a quart of milk a day prevents cancer. Bone meal retards aging.

And so on — all the way up to the present. We continue to seek the di-etary key to longevity and health. Today the trend is toward no-fat or low-fat foods.

The contemporary wisdom — and culture — condemning fat began in the 1970s. (Remember the model Twiggy?) In 1977, George McGovern's Select Committee on Nutrition and Human Needs announced that Amer-icans should cut back on fat. The committee's report, called "Dietary Goals for the United States," told us to cut down on cholesterol (a fat), other fats, and sugar. We were told to eat fiber-rich and cruciferous vegetables and fruit (such as broccoli, cabbage, and apples). Within ten years, at least ten more health agencies had provided similar advice.

At the same time, conflicting advice on the same subject began to proliferate. Dr. Robert Atkins, writer of many successful diet books in the 1970s, told people they could eat as much high-fat food as they wanted as long as they didn't eat carbohydrates, fruits, and vegetables. Then in 1981 Nathan Pritikin told consumers to cut fat to 10 percent, even though the government recommended a 30 percent intake. Recently Dr. Walter Willett of the Harvard School for Public Health told the *New York Times* (10 May 1995) that the famous government recommendation to limit fat intake to 30 percent in order to prevent heart disease isn't based on facts. Dr. Willett claimed that research hasn't identified an ideal amount of fat for our diets.

The "Seven Countries Study" of 1980, which has been considered the pivotal study for dietary recommendations, compared heart disease rates and dietary fat intake among different countries. The heart disease rate was lower where less fat was eaten. However, the lowest heart disease rate was found in Crete, where people ate 40 percent fat! A Harvard study showed that certain types of fat, such as olive oil, can help ward off cancer. It seems that the type of fat consumed, not simply the amount, is most important.

No wonder we're confused! What do we do? Should we simply eat, drink, and be merry, for tomorrow we die?

Virtually all ancient wisdom has prescribed *moderation* as an ideal path toward health. Fat isn't evil. We shouldn't be morbidly scared of it. Rather, a diet composed *only* of fat, or a diet without any fat at all, is what's dangerous. Our culture's obsession with fat has led to healthful changes and greater awareness in eating habits. There are areas of strong consensus among scientific studies, such as the benefits of eating fruits and vegetables, and the risks of eating too much fatty meat. Let's use our knowledge and also enjoy our lives: *intelligently* eating, drinking, and being merry.

And if you really crave a Big Mac (or movie theater popcorn fried in coconut oil), buy it, bite into it, and savor it. Maybe what we really need is research studies on the health benefits of *enjoying* food — the good, the bad, the fattening, and the low-fat alike.

# AIDS, FEAR, AND THE MIDDLE-CLASS HETEROSEXUAL

**H**eterosexuals have become so afraid of contracting AIDS that they lie awake at night in bed with their long-term heterosexual monogamous partner and worry whether that partner was monogamous five years earlier. A heterosexual hesitates to shake hands with an old friend who is now HIV-positive, even though HIV can't be transmitted just by shaking hands, and the HIV positive friend, who has already faced so much anguish, feels even more from being ostracized. A woman dies when she refuses a blood transfusion because she is afraid — unnecessarily — of tainted blood.

Why have we focused so much attention on the risk of heterosexual AIDS? Because the media told us we are in impending danger. As summarized in the *American Spectator*, July 1994, in 1994, CNN proclaimed that new AIDS cases rose 111 percent in 1993 "because of a sharp increase in infections among heterosexuals. . . . AIDS resulting from heterosexual contact in 1993 rose 130%." *Time* and *Newsweek*, always jumping at a sensational story, reported that AIDS cases had doubled in 1993 largely because of infections in heterosexuals. Even past surgeon general Antonia Novello said in the *Los Angeles Times* (as quoted in an article from *American Legion* magazine, September 1993) that "AIDS in homosexual men will be surpassed by AIDS in heterosexuals in some parts of the population."

The increased rate of heterosexual AIDS was reported in 1993 when the Centers for Disease Control expanded the definition of AIDS. Before 1993, an official diagnosis of the disease required that a person (1) was HIV-positive *and* (2) had symptoms typical of homosexuals in the later stages of AIDS. But in 1993, the CDC said that an official diagnosis of AIDS required only HIV-positive status and a blood T-cell count below two hundred. AIDS also could be officially diagnosed if an HIV-positive person had pulmonary tuberculosis, recurring pneumonia, or invasive cervical cancer, diseases much more common among heterosexuals than homosexuals.

Why is this important? The change in definition increased the number of people who would be counted as having AIDS. People who were HIV-positive but hadn't been officially diagnosed — such as women — became part of the AIDS statistics. The change also meant that people who wouldn't have joined the statistics under the earlier, narrower definitions for several more years suddenly became diagnosed with AIDS. In fact, as Michael Fumento reported in his book *The Myth of Heterosexual AIDS* (1993), if we compare 1993 to 1992 using the *original* definition, there was a 2 percent *decrease* in AIDS overall. Heterosexual cases were *slowing*, not increasing, by the original CDC definition. That's great news, but it was ignored by the media.

But why would the CDC change its definition, causing more grief and fear in everyone? The CDC changed its definition for two good reasons. The new definition meant that nonhomosexual AIDS sufferers could get the federal support and other benefits (such as free medication) that an official diagnosis of AIDS would bring them. Second, interest groups such as ACT UP had been pressuring the CDC to broaden the definition, both to help people receive benefits and also to keep the statistics high. These groups wanted to keep AIDS a "hot issue" so that research funding would continue. So for these reasons, the CDC expanded the definition of AIDS. It was great for treating sufferers of AIDS, but it seriously skewed the statistics for heterosexuals.

The reported *rate* of increase of AIDS among heterosexuals is also misleading. The horrified cries that we've been hearing about a "130% increase!" among heterosexuals make the spread of infection sound much worse than it truly is. Look more carefully at the numbers behind that "rate." We might hear that AIDS is increasing among heterosexuals at a rate of 130 percent, which is higher than the current rate among homosexuals. However, what that statement doesn't include is the fact that the heterosexual group is only a tiny fraction, in terms of actual size, of the other group (homosexuals). Let's simplify the math to see the problem more clearly. If there are 10 heterosexuals who have AIDS, and 10 more then come down with it, that's a 100 percent increase. But if there are 10,000 homosexuals who have AIDS, and then 1,000 more contract it, that's an increase of only 10 percent. The "100% increase among heterosexuals" sounds a lot worse than the "10% increase," doesn't it? But actually we're talking about 10 people versus 1,000.

All this attention to AIDS in the heterosexual middle class doesn't begin to describe who *really* has the disease! In 1994, the Centers for Disease Control released numbers on who really has AIDS, and how they got it:

- 54 percent were homosexual
- 24 percent were heterosexual but used drugs intravenously
- 2 percent were recipients of drug transfusions
- 1 percent were hemophiliacs
- 7 percent were homosexual and used drugs intravenously
- 6 percent didn't know how they got AIDS
- *only 6 percent (or 23,069 people) contracted AIDS through heterosexual contact*

As for that 6 percent who contracted AIDS through heterosexual contact, most had slept with an intravenous drug user (*Los Angeles Times,* 17 September 1994).

In spite of this reassurance, AIDS is nothing to scoff at. It deserves the personal concern and research dollars devoted to it. At the same time, worrying too much about AIDS — especially if you are not in a high-risk group — can cause more harm than good.

One of the worst results of the heterosexual AIDS paranoia is homophobia. When we become really frightened, we tend to run from the people who make us face those fears. Now the media have been screaming at us that heterosexuals are not immune to a disease many heterosexuals thought could only occur to "them." For some heterosexuals, that reality threatens to obscure sexual differences, and evokes fears of death. So what do some heterosexuals do when they feel the fear of AIDS? They blame, hate, slander, or fear homosexuals.

With AIDS, we must understand the real, and yet quite limited, risks for heterosexuals, and intelligently channel our energy and federal dollars toward the groups that are really suffering the most.

# THE SCARLET "H"

**J**oan and Kevin have been dating casually for a few weeks. They have a lot in common, including important values. Tonight they've had a romantic dinner at Joan's apartment. They each think that "tonight's the night" for their first time making love.

Still fully clothed, Kevin is on top of Joan on the couch, or is it Joan on top of Kevin? It's hard to tell because they're having so much fun. Suddenly Kevin stops, sits up, and says, "We should talk about our sexual histories." His words put a damper on their ardor, but Joan appreciates his desire to talk *before* they sleep together.

"Well," she starts, "I had genital warts a couple of years ago. And I had chlamydia once. They're both treated now." Both of these sexually transmitted diseases, she knows, are extremely common. The warts can recur anytime but haven't so far.

"I've never had those," Kevin says. "But I have herpes." Joan pulls away. She remembers reading a *Time* magazine story back in the mid-'80s about "the scarlet letter," H for herpes.

"It's not really a problem," Kevin is continuing. "I have an outbreak about twice a year, and I just don't have sex then. Pretty much the only way to pass herpes is during an outbreak."

" 'Pretty much?' " She thinks. How do either of them know she wouldn't get it?

"There's a tiny chance — maybe a few days a year — that you can get it through what they call 'asymptomatic shedding.' That's if the virus is on my skin without my knowing it. But if we use condoms, that shouldn't be a problem."

"*Always* use condoms?" Joan had been dreaming about marrying Kevin, and she wanted to have children. How could she have kids if they had to use condoms every time they had sex?

"Even if you do get it someday, it's not the end of the world. A herpes sore is just an annoyance. That's all. It doesn't lead anywhere else or cause other problems, like chlamydia or warts."

Joan stood up. "What do you mean 'it's not the end of the world'?! Speak for yourself!"

Should Joan refuse to sleep with Kevin because he has herpes? Should she be so afraid of this disease?

Herpes has received more overblown media attention than any other sexually transmitted disease until the discovery of AIDS. That media attention — and the panicked responses it evoked — have been responsible for countless stories of heartbreak. People who have herpes — and that's 1 in 4 people in the United States — can feel like no one will want them simply because they have this sexually transmitted disease.

Herpes is not actually one disease, it's a family of viruses, including herpes zoster and the herpes simplex virus (HSV). Herpes zoster causes chicken pox and shingles. HSV comes in two forms: HSV1 and HSV2. HSV1 typically produces cold sores around the mouth. HSV2 usually causes genital herpes. Both HSV viruses, however, can be spread from the mouth to the genitals.

Herpes does carry risks. An infected mother can transmit the infection to her infant. But that risk can be virtually eliminated if a pregnant woman lets her doctor know she has the disease. The doctor then can monitor the mother's condition, and if an outbreak occurs late in the pregnancy, he can prevent transmission through delivery by cesarean section. Studies are not yet conclusive, but at least one does suggest that HIV may be transmitted through genital blisters caused by HSV2.

Nevertheless, of all sexually transmitted diseases — gonorrhea, syphilis, chlamydia, genital warts (HPV, or human papillomavirus), and more — herpes is the most benign. All of the other diseases can lead to infertility and, in the case of genital warts, to cancer. Herpes leads to nothing else. The herpes viruses remain dormant in the body, like thousands of other viruses that we harbor, and travel to the infection site (such as the genitals) when the body's immune system is lower for whatever reason. The viruses cause a small, painful blister on the skin, but sometimes it is hardly noticeable. After a few days, even without treatment, the blister goes away. That's it.

Herpes is also incredibly common. Eighty percent of us suffer occasionally from herpes zoster, which emerges in the form of cold sores on the lips and/or nose. We don't socially ostracize people if they have a cold sore on their lips (which is passed the same way that genital herpes is passed, through direct contact). But we have ostracized people who happen to have these sores on their genitals.

Long-term research studies, such as the UCLA "Couples Study" in the 1980s, have shown that a person with herpes doesn't always transmit the disease to his or her partner, even if the couple isn't using condoms. Couples sleep together for years without the noninfected partner ever being infected with herpes.

Despite these facts, herpes has been elevated from the minor inconvenience that it is into a nightmare, raging disease. The media needed some dread disease to focus on in the mid-'80s (note that herpes coverage declined dramatically once the media had something really worth focusing on, AIDS). Herpes is more a media construction than a serious public health problem. And it is a "social disease" in the true sense of the word: the primary harm is social, not physical. Some people who contract herpes withdraw from dating altogether because they are afraid of rejection if they tell someone that they have the infection.

What people like this might not know is how many other people have herpes. The Herpes Resource Center of the American Social Health Association estimates that about 25 percent of the people in the United States (or sixty-five million) have genital herpes. That's far more than the entire population of Canada (which is twenty-eight million). Each year in the United States we have an estimated 500,000 new herpes infections.

Not all of these people know that they have herpes, and having herpes causes no problem for two-thirds of them. One-third of those who are infected with the virus never have outbreaks (they have built up strong antibodies). Another third have tiny outbreaks that they don't really notice. The remaining third have noticeable outbreaks like Kevin described.

Unlike some sexually transmitted diseases, herpes can be treated and even suppressed. Even the third of herpes carriers who do have outbreaks can prevent them by taking a drug called acyclovir. Acyclovir disables the herpes virus and for most people carries no side effects.

But herpes is *incurable* — right? That's right: in the same way that the common cold is incurable. Viruses continue to live in your body, and you develop antibodies to them. Unlike bacterial infections, which generally respond to antibiotics, viral infections are "incurable."

It's certainly wise to take precautions against the possibility of getting herpes. But it's certainly not worth breaking off a relationship with someone you love. And if you already have herpes (one-fourth of you do), your primary concern should be to educate other people to the reality of this "disease," rather than the horrors fabricated by the media blitz.

# EVERYTHING CAUSES CANCER

Sometimes it really does seem like everything causes cancer. A computerized search through various news media databases identifies literally thousands of stories on cancer and cancer-causing agents each year. We're all only too familiar with the headline: "... Causes Cancer." (You fill in the blank.)

It's true that cancer is the second-biggest killer in the United States, after heart disease. It certainly makes sense to wonder what has caused this increase in cancer deaths. Cancer kills more than half a million Americans annually. Heart disease, though, kills 40 percent more — 700,000 people — but gets much less press.

Here is a litany of only some of the many carcinogens presented to us as explanations for the rise in cancer: smoking, secondhand smoke, dioxin, Alar, DDT, asbestos, nuclear power, electromagnetic fields, radon, benzene, air pollution, radiation and X rays, ultraviolet rays, food dyes, tanning beds, breast implants, red meat, saccharine, coffee, insecticides sprayed by crop dusters in Third World countries, water, chinaware, paint, video display terminals, cell phones, any packaged food, pesticides in general. . . .

Notice that all of these alleged carcinogens are products of industrialization, or at least weren't identified as causing cancer until we had developed sophisticated technology (in the case of radon and other gases, for example). The arrival of these products and elements of industrialization into our lives has coincided with the increase in cancer. We have connected the two: the incidence of cancer has risen along with industrialization. Therefore, many have concluded, the products of industrialization *cause* cancer. This is a convenient explanation.

What is usually not presented to us, though, is the No. 1 cause of cancer: old age. Old age has also "increased," so to speak, throughout the twentieth century. We can now expect to live past the age of seventy-five. In 1900, we lived only half that long. As Bruce Ames, chief of the Microbial Genetics Section at the prestigious National Institutes of Health, pointed out in an interview with the *Los Angeles Times* (11 August 1994), "The incidence of cancer goes up very sharply with age. Mice live two years; by the end of their life span about a third of them have cancer. Monkeys live twenty or thirty years; by the end of their life span about a third of them have cancer. People live eighty or ninety years; by the end of our life span, about a third of us have cancer." In other words, cancer in old age is not abnormal at all. There's nothing to blame but old age itself.

Columnist Robert Scheer explains that "longevity is the real epidemic, the greatest danger to our health. Because we live longer, we are more likely to develop health problems associated with aging that our shorter-lived great-grandparents didn't face" (*Playboy*, March 1995). Ames phrases the same idea slightly differently: "Now that we've conquered all those diseases, we're living long enough to get cancer."

Ames explains why old age predisposes a person to cancer. Our metabolism is based upon oxygen, and the by-products of oxygen cause infinitesimal "lesions" in each of our cells each day. These lesions also can harm the DNA in cells. When those cells divide, as our cells do continuously, any harm to the DNA is passed on. Ames says that "by the time you're old, we find a few million oxygen lesions per cell. And when the cell divides, those turn into mutations, or some percentage of them does. Most mutations don't matter, but some are in key genes and then you have cancer."

There's not a lot we can do about our need for oxygen. But by increasing our dietary intake of antioxidants — such as Vitamin C, carotenoids, and Vitamin E — we can combat some of the negative effects of oxygen on our cells. Dr. Gladys Block of the University of California at Berkeley has found strong evidence that eating fruits and vegetables (the best sources of antioxidants) protects us from cancer. Dr. Block analyzed 172 epidemiological studies from around the world to arrive at this conclusion.

Perhaps our improved diets — more fruits and veggies — can account for the lower cancer rate that we've seen recently. (Yes, *lower*, despite the media hype about carcinogens everywhere.) In fact, as our population is aging, we actually have less cancer than we would expect. People live longer, so we should see more cases of cancer, right? Wrong.

The Centers for Disease Control tell us that death rates for most forms of cancer have been declining for decades. Sixty years ago, cancer of the stomach killed just over 31 people out of every 100,000. Today cancer of the stomach kills fewer than 5 in 100,000. Because pap smears and other gynecological cancer prevention tests are so widespread, uterine cancer has declined from 31 cases per 100,000 to 6. Liver cancer has seen a similar striking drop (*Los Angeles Times*, 11 September 1994).

The exceptions to this general decline are lung cancer and leukemia (cancer of the blood). Twice as many people today (6 in 100,000) die from leukemia than in the 1930s, and almost twelve times as many die from lung cancer. Sixty years ago, lung cancer killed only 3 people in every 100,000, while now it kills about 48. Lung cancer is believed to be caused almost entirely by smoking.

The media furor over preventing cancer is useful in some respects. News reports tell us that smoking does indeed cause cancer. Living directly underneath a high-power electrical line could cause cancer. Pesticides do cause cancer, at least in the high quantities given to laboratory animals. High levels of radon in a closed room can cause cancer. And so on.

More than anything else, cancer has become the symbol of our mortality. No wonder, then, that we obsess over it, seek to explain it away, try to overcome it, hate it, and fear it. Amazingly, our advancing technology is managing to understand and control it, at least somewhat. We shouldn't be scaring ourselves to death over cancer, but thanking our scientists and physicians for allowing us to live longer and for making inroads in prevention and treatment of this dreaded disease.

# "PESTICIDES PREVENT CANCER"
# (NO, THAT'S NOT A TYPO)

**W**hat? Isn't this title wrong? Shouldn't it read "Pesticides *Cause* Cancer"? That's what headlines of news stories across the nation have shouted to us for years now. "Pesticides Levels Unsafe for Children." "Toxic Strawberries." "Is Your Family Safe?"

No, the title "Pesticides Prevent Cancer" is correct. This chapter will show you not only that synthetic pesticides are safe (as currently regulated by the government) in our diets, but that their existence actually does help keep us healthier.

We can discover some of the reasons for optimism by following the story of one of the world's most famous and respected biochemists, Dr. Bruce Ames. Dr. Ames started as a critic of pesticides and, through his illustrious career, has become a champion of the benefits of pesticides. First, here are his credentials. Ames is chief of the Microbial Genetics Section of the National Institutes of Health, chairman of the Biochemistry Department at the University of California, Berkeley, and a member of the National Academy of Sciences. Other honors include service on the Board of Directors of the National Cancer Institute, numerous scientific awards, and over three hundred scientific papers in prestigious journals. He is currently the director of the National Institute of Environmental Health Sciences Center. He does no work for private industry that could lead him to make "scientific" pronouncements that support a commercial purpose more than a scientific one.

Early in his career, Dr. Ames was the darling of environmentalists and an outspoken critic of pesticides and man-made food additives. Today, fifteen years later, Dr. Ames says, "Unless you wade around in the stuff, pesticides don't cause cancer. That's the bottom line!" (*Forbes*, 25 October 1993) In fact, he thinks that pesticides help *prevent* cancer.

What happened during those fifteen years? Dr. Ames invented a sophisticated test to determine the cancer-causing potential of various substances — from chemical pesticides to dyes to foods. The test identified the presence of "mutagens," which cause cancer. As a result of his tests, many synthetics were indeed identified as carcinogenic and were pulled off the market.

However, what Dr. Ames and his colleagues also found was that mutagens are everywhere — in supposedly benign, "natural" foods as well as in synthetic pesticides. As Dr. Ames explained, "There were mutagens in celery and in a cup of coffee. The natural world is full of mutagens." Peanut butter contains aflatoxin, a known carcinogen. Many spices, smoked or salted fish, corn, pickled dishes, and broiled or fried beef, pork, eggs, and chicken are only a few other "natural" foods that contain cancer-causing mutagens.

As a result of these findings, Dr. Ames began to look more critically at the antipesticide environmental movement. He saw that this movement tended to divide all foods and substances into two camps: " 'If it's man-made, it's bad; if it's natural, it's fine.' " He explains, "That didn't fit with anything I knew about toxicology, so I became increasingly suspicious of this kind of thing."

Just because a substance is synthetic or man-made doesn't mean that it will cause cancer. Conversely, just because a substance is "natural" doesn't mean that it's not a carcinogen. Dr. Ames is fond of pointing out that a cup of coffee contains ten milligrams of natural carcinogens, which is about how much pesticide residue the average person ingests in a year. Eating a full year's worth of nonorganic produce, then, is as dangerous as drinking one cup of coffee.

So maybe buying fruits and vegetables at the nonorganic market isn't so dangerous after all. Actually, quite the opposite. Many studies have proven that consumption of fresh fruits and vegetables is one of our best *preventions* for cancer. Dr. Ames claims today that "pesticides lower cancer rates because they make fruits and vegetables cheaper and people buy more of them." Hundreds of studies have proven that eating fruits and vegetables, with their antioxidant Vitamins A, C, and E, is our best defense against cancer.

But what do we read about in the news? The synthetic carcinogens are all around us. In 1992, researchers Robert Lichter, Stanley Rothman, and Mark Mills analyzed 1,147 news stories on cancer that had been published over the last twenty years. These researchers saw that the media paid the most attention to artificial carcinogens, most of which scientists think are low-risk.

At the same time, the media tended to ignore the many "natural" carcinogens around us.

Dr. Ames also presents us with a different way of looking at pesticides. He points out that we eat "pesticides," in the literal sense, in every bite we take of any food that comes from the earth. "Pesticides" are like plants' immune systems. Plants don't have weapons to ward off insects, and if plants hadn't developed natural chemical "pesticides," they would have been devoured by insects and become extinct millennia ago. Dr. Ames said that "99.99% of the pesticides we consume are naturally present in plants to ward off insects and other predators." We ingest ten thousand times more natural pesticides than artificial pesticide residues every day.

The real danger of all the media attention paid to synthetic pesticides is that more-serious problems are ignored. Daniel Puzo, who covers food safety for the *Los Angeles Times*, has pointed out that all the attention to pesticides — and the research money thrown into it — have meant that government and the public haven't focused on more dangerous risks, such as bacteria-borne food illnesses (including salmonella and *E. coli* bacteria). According to the Centers for Disease Control, the United States reports 6.5 million food-borne illnesses per year, with nine thousand deaths from food poisoning. This is a much higher rate than cancers allegedly caused by pesticides, but we don't hear about them.

Elizabeth Whelan, president of the American Council on Science and Health (a consumer-education organization), thinks that consumers who choose organic produce make this choice based more on fear than on reason. She states (*New York Times*, 7 July 1995) that people get confused over the pesticide risk issue, merging "real concerns with hypothetical ones." If the pesticide risk is 1 in 1 million, while the risk of bacterial contamination in food is 1 in 100,000, people might still focus on pesticides.

There are dozens more encouraging testimonials about pesticide safety that we could report here. We'll briefly mention a couple more to encourage you to eat fruits and vegetables in peace and confidence.

The University of California at Davis FoodSafe Program provides research-based information concerning food safety to the public, educators, and regulatory agencies. Dr. Carl Winter, the program's director, cites the Food and Drug Administration's "Total Diet Study," in which researchers purchased food at retail outlets, cooked or prepared it as we normally do, and then analyzed the pesticide levels. The FDA found that our average exposure to pesticide residues is less than 1 percent of the level that is "allowable" — that is, safe levels "based on the results of long-term animal toxicology studies and conservative 'safety factors.'"

In a report titled "Pesticides and Food Safety: Doing the Right Thing for the Wrong Reasons," Dr. Winter reviewed a National Academy of Sciences study that, he says, "concluded that the significant health benefits from consumption of a diet rich in fruits and vegetables (such as decreases in heart disease and in certain types of cancer) far outweigh any potential risks from pesticide residues in the diet. In a recent California consumer survey performed by a UC Davis colleague, however, 8 percent of consumers surveyed made the unhealthy choice to decrease their consumption of produce due to pesticide concerns." This fear-based behavior isn't protecting us; rather, we're scaring ourselves to death.

What about the impact of pesticides on children and infants, whose bodies are more immature and vulnerable? Dr. Winter points out another National Academy of Sciences report, titled "Pesticides in the Diets of Infants and Children" (1993). Although the Academy found serious deficiencies in the methods used to assess risks and regulate pesticide use for children and infants, the report nevertheless told parents to continue to feed children lots of fruits and vegetables. The benefits of fresh produce far outweighed the risks.

The American Cancer Society, the American Medical Association, the World Health Organization, and many other scientific groups have gone on record that they aren't worried about the risks from pesticide residues in our diet. What we should be concerned about, these organizations all say, is problems of microbial contamination (such as E. *coli* or salmonella), and most of all the need to eat a nutritionally balanced diet, including fruits and vegetables, which the careful use of pesticides has made more readily available to the public.

All of the media attention paid to pesticides has proven to be a double-edged sword. It has been bad because fear of cancer-causing pesticides has kept people from eating fresh produce, the very thing that prevents cancer. On the other hand, the attention has been good because pesticides *can* cause cancer if they are found in high amounts on food. The media hype has led to tighter regulations on pesticide use, which affects not only our food, but our groundwater, our atmosphere, and the health of farm workers.

Several federal agencies are intensely involved in pesticide regulation, including the Environmental Protection Agency, the Food and Drug Administration, and the Department of Agriculture, all the way up to the president's office. For example, the EPA is busy considering how to improve the measurement of pesticides in our food. Procedures are being developed to check not how much pesticide is on the produce as it leaves the farm (which is how pesticides are currently measured) but how much actually makes it to the dinner plate. Pesticide residue can sometimes be reduced by washing the produce; other times the pesticides become more concentrated by the methods used in preparing processed foods. The plan would also consider the impact of pesticides on children, who have immature bodies and consume more fruits and vegetables in proportion to body weight than adults do.

The trend is toward toughening pesticide regulations. In 1949, the FDA set the first safety standard for food additives, and then tightened it in 1960 with the "Delaney Clause," which requires a "zero-risk" standard. Because today we have sensitive chemical methods for identifying truly minuscule quantities of carcinogens — in parts per billion or trillion — the EPA has been allowing "negligible risk" for small amounts of pesticide. However, in October 1994 the Clinton administration signed an agreement to uphold the Delaney Clause. This agreement means that up to eighty-five popular pesticides could be banned, but with the ban phased in over five years so that farmers can find substitutes.

Weighing the pros and cons, clearly pesticides are a positive result of chemical technology. They make fresh fruits and vegetables plentiful and readily available. Other biochemical technology allows government and private-interest agencies to become "watchdogs" to make sure that pesticides don't go awry. Bite into the apple, make a strawberry pie, steam some zucchini, cut into a cantaloupe, toss a salad, eat your brussels sprouts — because you can hardly do anything better for your health.

# HAMBURGERS: THE ALL-AMERICAN . . . POISON?

In 1994, every American ate an estimated sixty-seven pounds of beef, on average. That means that America consumed almost *seventeen billion pounds of beef* in 1994 alone. And hamburgers are about as all-American a form of beef as you can get. They're the centerpieces in barbecues all across the United States, shared by people in New England, the Old South, the Midwest, the Great Plains, sunny California, the western deserts, and even the Pacific Northwest. All over the world people are eating Big Macs. Almost everyone loves hamburgers.

So what happens when hamburgers *kill* people?

In the fall of 1993, four children died and over seven hundred people became seriously ill from eating hamburgers at Jack in the Box fast food restaurants along the Pacific coast. The burgers, it turned out, had been made with meat contaminated with "E. coli 0157:H7" bacteria. At the time the bacteria were little known, but we soon learned that it is extremely aggressive. Individuals who are already somewhat vulnerable to disease, such as the elderly, children, and pregnant women, are this bacteria's favorite victims. The bacteria slowly shuts down all of a person's vital organs, one after another, until the person dies. That's what happened to the four children.

Later, it was discovered that the contaminated meat had not been heated to the recommended internal temperature of 155 degrees Fahrenheit. But federal officials, such as experts from the Centers for Disease Control, the Food and Drug Administration, and the Department of Agriculture, never could figure out exactly where the *E. coli* bacteria had entered the system. Was it in the slaughterhouse? During the grinding process? In transport? In the Jack in the Box outlet, where food workers may have left the beef unrefrigerated, or perhaps hadn't cooked it long enough?

Experts say this crisis could happen again. As the Institute for Science in Society said in a study reported in the *Los Angeles Times* (22 September 1994), "Bacterial contamination of meat and poultry is a time bomb waiting to go off." In fact, *E. coli* outbreaks occurred again in California in 1994, although not with the severity of 1993. This time, three children were hospitalized.

Should you be scared about eating a hamburger at a fast-food restaurant or at a baseball game? How about the meat at the grocery store? How do we know what's safe?

The answer, happily, is that you can still enjoy hamburgers, even at fast-food restaurants. Sometimes a company will use a crisis to examine its operations and make meaningful improvements. That's what Jack in the Box did — and they created a new standard and system for food safety that has been copied around the world.

Jack in the Box and most large restaurant chains have adopted a program called the Hazard Analysis Critical Control Point program, which locates and monitors all of the critical points in the food system where the integrity of their products might be compromised, including processing, transportation, cooking, and serving. This program was originally created in the 1960s for the space program to ensure that the astronauts' food was sterile. This system exceeds the standards set by the U.S. Food and Drug Administration for safe food processing, transport, preparation, and service.

Let's assume that one-third of the beef consumed in the United States in 1994 went into hamburgers — about 5.3 billion pounds — and that hamburgers are made with a quarter-pound of beef each. That year alone, then, Americans consumed over twenty-one billion hamburgers. In 1993 fewer than eight hundred made people sick. That is still too many, but with tighter inspections of beef processing plants, better testing methods, and higher standards in the fast-food industry, even these minimal risks should decrease.

# MAD AS A . . . COW?!?

"Killed by Mad Cow Disease"
— Headline in the *New Statesman & Society,* 29 March 1996

"Silence of the Calves"
— Headline in the *Economist,* 6 April 1996

"Mad Cow Epidemic Puts Spotlight on Puzzling Human Brain Disease"
— Headline in the *New York Times,* 2 April 1996

"Fatal Case in France"
— Headline in the *New York Times,* 27 April 1996

Judging from these and other headlines in the early part of 1996, you would think that the human race faces a devastating epidemic. True, it is a devastating disease in cows, and thus affects the beef and cattle industry financially, but to worry that "mad cow" disease is a real threat to the human population is a bit of a stretch.

What needs to be cleared up, though, is that bovine spongiform encephalopathy (BSE) — commonly labeled "mad cow" disease — is a cattle disease. The observable symptoms during the final stages of the disease are easily recognized. These include abnormal gait, increased sensitivity, loss of coordination, and in a minority of cattle the aggression that earned the disease its popular name (*Science,* 247:523, 1990).

BSE, scrapie, and Creutzfeldt-Jakob disease (CJD) are neurodegenerative diseases of cattle, sheep, and humans respectively. All are characterized by long incubation periods, over ten years in many cases, before onset of any clinical symptoms. Unlike typical viral and bacterial infections, the infecting "agent" in these diseases is a protein (called a "prion"), but a small, still-undiscovered helper-virus might also be involved (*Scientific American*, August 1990). In about 15 percent of all CJD cases a specific, inherited mutation is to blame for the disease (*Science*, 271:1798, 1996). Kuru, which is similar to CJD and was first discovered in New Guinea, was shown to be transmitted by ritualistic handling and eating of human brain, an activity few modern people are likely to practice.

BSE was first identified in November 1986 in Britain. Most scientists believe that the spread of the disease was facilitated by the common practice of feeding meat and bone meal in rations to cattle as a source of protein. This practice, however, became widespread in the 1920s, so how come it is only ten years since BSE was first noticed? The reason may lie in the fact that up until the early '80s, an organic solvent (e.g., chloroform and acetone, also known as nail polish remover) extraction step, used to extract tallow from sheep and other animal carcasses in the production of cattle feed, was excluded and replaced by heat treatment. Ironically, the "infectious agent" in BSE is destroyed by organic solvents, but can withstand temperatures above that of boiling water (*New Scientist*, October 1993). Eight years later nearly 150,000 animals on over 30,000 British farms had the disease (*New Scientist*, February 1995).

So what has all this to do with BSE, and how come humans are catching a cattle disease? To start with, no one has shown conclusively that BSE can be transmitted to humans through eating beef. However, an article in the highly regarded journal *Lancet* (April 6, 1996) presents data that show a possible link with BSE in ten patients with CJD-like symptoms. Worldwide CJD occurs in about 1 person per 1 million per year. In western countries many of those cases can be traced to tissues taken from (infected) cadavers and used in specialized surgery, or hormones produced from the pituitary glands of diseased people (*Scientific American*, August 1990).

Mass hysteria has decimated the British beef industry to the point where some are calling for the slaughtering of all cattle in the United Kingdom. Only a few BSE cases have been reported in Europe outside the United Kingdom, and inspectors in the United States are tracking down a handful of cattle that were imported before BSE was commonly identified. Over the next decade or so new BSE cases are certain to decrease dramatically, due to the new regulations that now prohibit feeding meat and bone meal to cattle. For those still worried, eating beef is still safe, just stay away from the offal from cattle, such as the brain, thymus, and spleen (BSE target organs). Keep in mind that you are more likely to choke on a bite of beef than to catch mad cow disease from it. So enjoy your juicy steak . . . but chew carefully!

## NIGHT OF THE LIVING FLESH-EATING SLIME . . .

When a newspaper headline sounds like the title of a horror movie, it's time to take a skeptical look at the claims of the story. A good example is the recent "flesh-eating bacteria" scare.

Headlines in Great Britain read "Killer Bug Ate My Face," "Eaten Alive," "Curse of the Killer Bacteria," and "Dither — and You Die." In the United States, *Time* magazine (12 September 1994) ran an eight-page article with two-inch type screaming, "The Killers All Around." *Time*'s story began, "They can strike anywhere, anytime. On a cruise ship, in the corner restaurant, in the grass just outside the back door. And anyone can be a carrier . . . even the sweetheart who seems perfect in every way. . . ."

Reading those words, did you run to the pharmacy to stock up on bandages and antibiotic ointment? Did you call the pediatrician to ask if your child could play outside with a scraped knee? Did you stay home from work with a minor sore throat, *just in case?* In other words, did you *not* live your life as fully as you could because of a negligible risk sensationalized by the media?

No, you might say, pointing to the article in the newspaper: this disease is for real. It's common — a cousin to the bacteria that causes strep throat — and it kills. The British "epidemic" of early 1994 killed a whopping eleven people (*Newsweek*, 20 June 1994). A few cases cropped up over summer 1994 across the United States, with several more reported in Great Britain. A college president in California was eaten alive by the bacteria. It struck him down within two days following a "misdiagnosis" from a doctor! The bacteria often infects a minor wound, which causes pain and fever. Then it starts killing, or "eating," the skin, penetrating through a sore or cut, and begins to gorge on the body. It leaves a trail of blackened dead tissue or, even worse, a gaping hole. It moves as fast as one inch per hour. It can kill in one day.

All this is true. It is *also* true that truth taken out of context, or reported only partially, is a lie.

The Centers for Disease Control in Atlanta report about five to fifteen hundred cases of severe streptococcus infection in the United States annually. Of these, less than 10 percent developed into a case of flesh-eating bacteria, or "necrotising fasciitus." (The term means literally "the dying of fascia," which is the tissue that connects muscles and skin.) The population of the United States is 258,245,000 — making the incidence of flesh-eating bacteria less than 1 in 2.5 million, or .0000003 percent.

And why is it that our well-paid researchers and doctors don't know much about this deadly disease? Is it because it's so mysterious and defies medical technology? No. Even though the disease has a long history — descriptions of it date back to 1783 in France — it occurs quite rarely. Scientists just don't have much chance to study it.

Necrotising fasciitus is caused by a bacteria that is in the same family as the bacteria that causes strep throat. You've had strep throat. Is the next logical step developing necrotising fasciitus? No. Just because you've harbored the bacteria that potentially causes the disease does not mean that you will come down with the disease.

While necrotising fasciitus is technically the same bacteria that causes strep throat, the two strains are different in the way that two types of apples might be different — a Granny Smith and a Golden Delicious, for example. "Group A beta-hemolytic streptococcus" is the deadlier, invasive, and genetically different strain of plain old strep A. Necrotising fasciitis occurs in 5 to 10 percent of cases of this more-severe form of strep. But strep bacteria, like other organisms, appears in a number of slightly different forms. In fact, *friendly* forms of streptococcus live happily in the bodies of about 25 percent of us, and we don't know that they're permanent house guests. Will these house guests turn into murderers of their host? Not likely.

If a house guest wanted to murder you, he or she would need a moment of opportunity. With necrotising fasciitus, the first condition is the presence of the highly rare bacterial strain to begin with. Then you need an open cut or sore to allow the killer bug to enter. (That's why children with chicken pox are more likely to contract it — although the risk is still extremely tiny. The bug can enter through the open sores caused by chicken pox.) If you don't have a cut or sore, or if you keep your wounds very clean, the bug is turned away at the door.

What's more, even if you are the 1 in 2.5 million who does contract the disease, it won't necessarily kill or maim you. If a person seeks medical attention within a couple of hours after developing symptoms, neither life nor limbs will be lost. The symptoms are strong: severe soreness, redness, and spreading swelling; high fever; and blistering of the skin.

Therefore, from without and within — in terms of the incidence of the disease in the overall population, and the precise conditions required inside the body — the probability that you will witness the spectacle of flesh-eating bacteria devouring your belly is about as likely as the chance that you will star in a hit horror flick and win an Academy Award.

Dr. Edward Kaplan of the University of Minnesota, who runs a World Health Organization laboratory responsible for tracking the strep germ, admits that we have an incomplete understanding of the strep bacteria, but still feels angry at the overblown media coverage of this bacteria. "If I lived in your part of the country," he told a reporter at the *Los Angeles Times* (15 June 1994), "I would be much more worried about an earthquake than I would about getting flesh-eating bacteria."

We love to fear flesh-eating bacteria for the same reasons that we thrill to the terror of horror movies. The British medical journal *Lancet* (19 November 1994) "reviewed" the latest horror queen star — necrotising fasciitus — in its article "Superbug Stars in Media-Made Epidemic." If this flesh-eating superstar enters your nightmares, just remember that she's much smaller in reality than she looks on the silver screen or in blown-up tabloid photos.

# HAUNTED BY HANTA

**K**iller rats! Mysterious plague spreads across the West!

Are these headlines from medieval Europe? The bubonic plague wiped out so many people that there weren't enough left to bury the dead. This plague was carried by rats. The now-famous "hantavirus" of 1993 brings up echoes of the plague, even though only thirty-two people were killed (versus millions in the bubonic plague) (*Morbidity and Mortality Weekly Report*, 13 May 1994). But as we've seen with other "scares," numbers and probability don't usually keep us from becoming scared anyway.

We all know that rodents carry disease, not only rabies, but a host of fearsome horrors. We scurry away from mice and rats with good reason. One of the latest of these horrors to enter our awareness was the hantavirus "plague" during the summer of 1993. When the hantavirus hit the headlines, we scurried far, far away from the area hardest hit — the "Four Corners" region of the United States, where New Mexico, Colorado, Arizona, and Utah meet.

Of course, people don't run away from a region of the country that has an unusually high traffic accident rate, even though traffic accidents claim far more lives than the hantavirus ever will. People don't even stay away from San Francisco or New York City because their AIDS rates are higher than those of the rest of the nation. So why all the uproar over hantavirus?

As the *Los Angeles Times* stated in an 11 June 1993 story on hantavirus, the disease "illustrates the potential for the emergence of deadly new infectious agents." That certainly grabs our attention, even though the hantavirus had existed a long time before being identified and named. Europe and Asia have experienced hantavirus outbreaks since the 1930s. Some United Nations troops were infected during the Korean War, and U.S. military personnel in Korea have also battled the disease. Cases of hantavirus have been reported sporadically for years in the United States: a case in 1980 in California, a single case each year in 1990 and 1991, and six cases in 1992 before the outbreak in 1993.

The hantavirus is frightening because it's a mystery illness that seems at first like a bad flue — fever, muscle aches, headache, red eyes — and then, sometimes within a few hours, causes death as the lungs fill with fluid. From New Mexico, the hantavirus "spread" to fourteen states.

The hantavirus, which takes its name from the Hanta Valley, where it was first identified, is also scary because scientists have a hard time isolating the strains of this virus. We're accustomed to scientists "mapping" a virus quickly, but this one is difficult to grow in a laboratory. In fact, one of the earlier strains of hantavirus took thirty years to grow in a lab.

If this virus is so tough to grow, how does it spread? According to the federal government's *Morbidity and Mortality Weekly Report* (30 July 1993), people contract the virus by breathing dust and other airborne particles from the saliva, feces, and urine of infected rodents. A bite from a rodent carrier can also lead to hantavirus infection. Eating food or drinking water contaminated with the virus can also bring it on.

The outbreak in 1993 occurred because of an explosion in the rodent population in the rural areas that were affected. Because of heavy rains in the previous year, the number of deer mice, the virus's favorite carrier, grew by ten times the normal population. Of the fifty-one cases reported, half were American Indians, mostly from the Navajo reservation. As a result of the outbreak, Congress authorized $6 million to keep the virus from spreading further. This money was spent mostly on informing people about ways to keep rodents out of their houses.

The hantavirus is relatively easy to prevent by proper sanitation and cleanliness. The hantavirus dies when it comes into contact with soap or household disinfectants, so rural dwellers also can avoid breathing hantavirus-contaminated dust by washing dishes immediately and by keeping surfaces clean. Other precautions include storing food (including pet food) in tightly sealed containers, keeping garbage in rodent-proof containers, sealing all openings through which rodents can enter the home, and setting rodent traps in woodpiles and unoccupied structures such as barns and storage sheds.

For most of us, and especially urbanites, the dangers of hantavirus are minuscule. (No, cats and dogs don't carry hantavirus.) For those living in rural areas, keeping the mouse out of the house is the best protection. Hantavirus is *not* the next bubonic plague.

# JUST A SMOKE SCREEN?

## NO SMOKING ALLOWED

The signs are everywhere: on the job, in public buildings, and increasingly in restaurants and even bars in many parts of the country. Nonsmokers have become increasingly intolerant of their nicotine-loving brethren. In many places, smokers have become near-pariahs. But is the danger from "secondhand smoke" real?

The courts and public officials seem to think so. Parents have lost child custody cases because they smoke. No one is allowed to smoke on domestic airline flights in the United States (there are no more "smoking sections"). Smoking is not allowed in over 30 percent of American workplaces. Nor is it allowed in restaurants in Los Angeles, California. Hillary Rodham Clinton has insisted that no one smoke in the White House. Even fast-food restaurants, including McDonald's, Taco Bell, and Jack in the Box, have prohibited smoking. The federal Occupational Safety and Health Administration is considering banning smoking in *all* workplaces.

Nevertheless, some people say that all the hoopla over secondhand smoke is just a smoke screen. Let's investigate the supposed dangers of secondhand smoke to see if this one, like many of the "risks" in our society, is more hype than truth.

Secondhand smoke wasn't seen as much of a risk until an Environmental Protection Agency report in 1993 declared it a "Group A" human carcinogen. The report said that secondhand smoke accounts for fifty-three thousand deaths each year, including three thousand from lung cancer. Actually, this piece of data was buried in the middle of the report, but the media made it a headline. *U.S. News and World Report* demanded on its cover, "Should Cigarettes Be Outlawed?" *Time* posed a daring question on its cover: "Is It All Over for Smokers?"

Good questions. Unfortunately, the answers weren't explored fully in the media — because the answers aren't all that clear. The media, particularly television, like clear-cut stories. This one is still shrouded in behind-the-scenes controversy.

Several hundred scientific studies have linked heavy secondhand smoke to diseases such as cancer, heart disease, respiratory infections, asthma, and sudden infant death syndrome (SIDS). The strongest link by far is to lung cancer. However, the relationship between secondhand smoke and the other diseases is far from established. Of the 53,000 deaths supposedly caused by secondhand smoke, most (37,000) were related to heart disease, and 12,000 to cancers other than lung cancer. Scientists do not agree about secondhand smoke and heart disease. Out of these several hundred studies, only fourteen were able to conclude that the link exists (*Los Angeles Times*, 26 May 1994).

Another question is how *much* smoke is "heavy" smoke. A third murky area is *just how much* secondhand smoke actually contributes to these diseases. And does it *cause* the disease, *worsen* a condition that was already brewing, or neither of the above?

Uncertainty among specialists is the only thing that is really clear about the majority of alleged deaths from secondhand smoke. The *Los Angeles Times* quotes one of the world's leading epidemiologists, Sir Richard Doll of Oxford University, who found that "there is a real problem estimating the quantitative effect of environmental tobacco smoke." Sheryl Stolberg, the *Los Angeles Times* (26 May 1994) medical writer, assessed the secondhand smoke issue this way: "A little bit of science — still emerging, not all of it conclusive — shaping a lot of public policy."

So why has secondhand smoke become such a captivating public issue? It has the word *cancer* associated with it, and that always gets lots of attention. The tobacco lobby and its opponents both have invested so much money and energy into the issue that they've heightened the controversy beyond where it might otherwise be. And the issue allows us to vent anger at the people we love to hate: the big tobacco companies. The tobacco companies are believed to have lied for so long about the risks of smoking, which they still deny, that vengeance is sweet.

ARE WE SCARING OURSELVES TO DEATH?        **77**

It seems quite clear that "heavy" secondhand smoke (define that however you want) can possibly lead to lung cancer. Is living with a smoker like a ticket to chemotherapy? Maybe, but a lot of people have lived with heavy smokers and not had problems. Will a whiff from someone's Marlboro down the hall give you cancer — or pose enough of a risk that you should deny that person the right to smoke in the hall? Probably not. It may be sensible to reduce or even prohibit smoking in offices and other enclosed spaces. However, the effort to vilify smokers and prevent virtually all smoking everywhere does seem to be an overreaction to the threats of secondhand smoke as we currently understand them.

# HOME SWEET
# HOME?

# THERE'S NO PLACE LIKE HOME

**H**ousehold Materials May Be Toxic, A Study Warns," says a *New York Times* (15 March 1995) headline. A picture labeled "Dangers in the Home" takes us on a tour of the dangers lurking within our four walls: toxic dry cleaning solution, chloroform in tap water, ammonia and other substances in cleaners, pesticides, lead in old pipes and paint, formaldehyde in particle board and carpeting, asbestos in the walls. . . . Aren't we even safe in our own homes?

"A man's home is his castle," the saying goes. Home is supposed to be the place where we retreat from the stresses and dangers of the outside world. But newspaper and evening news headlines lead us to wonder whether our homes are turning into nightmares. How about the video display terminals on our televisions and computers — do those cause cancer? Do the electrical wires outside our windows emit electromagnetic fields that cause birth defects? Does the dishware in our cabinets give us lung cancer by shedding radon?

We are scaring ourselves to death in our own homes. How grounded are all these fears? This section critically examines several alleged dangers in our homes. After reading this section you should be able to rest easier at night in your own bed, breathe easier in your own rooms, make wiser decisions about your home environment, and enjoy life just a bit more.

# RADIOACTIVE DISHES?
# RADON IN THE HOME

Y ou're curled up in front of the television after a long day at work. You've scooped some ice cream into one of your grandmother's vintage Fiesta bowls, the ones you inherited. Fiesta dishware pieces are collectors' items, particularly the ones with the original bright orange glaze, like your grand-mother's. You like the way your favorite vanilla ice cream looks against the orange.

You're watching the evening news when suddenly you become aware that the report you're hearing is talking about your grandmother's dishes. "The top-selling dishware in U.S. history, the original Fiesta ware, can cause lung cancer," the newscaster intones. *What?* He continues: "In particular it is the orange Fiesta ware made before 1972 that is potentially carcinogenic." Great, you think, as you set aside the ice cream in your orange bowl and turn up the volume. Is *nothing* safe?

The newscaster explains that the bright orange glaze in Fiesta ceramics is uranium-based and not only emits gamma rays, which apparently has been known for decades, but also releases radon, a gas that causes lung cancer. A single Fiesta plate in an unventilated, average-size room can produce more than seven times the radioactive radon gas that has been deemed safe by the government. The radon escapes through cracks in the glaze — cracks so tiny that they're not visible to the naked eye.

According to a report in the *Los Angeles Times* (23 April 1994), about 200 million Fiesta ware pieces in a variety of colors have been sold since the company introduced the dishware line in 1936. The uranium-based orange glaze was used until 1972, except between 1943 and 1959, when the government placed restrictions on the use of uranium. In 1976 the company reintroduced the Fiesta line, but without the lead- and uranium-based orange glazes. The new orange color isn't quite the same as the old, which is why the older orange Fiesta plates are such collectors' items. The old dishes are safe to collect, as long as they're stored or displayed in a well-ventilated room. However, people shouldn't eat off of them, the Food and Drug Administration advises.

You get up from your comfortable chair and open a window, even though it's cold outside. Is there too much radon in the room? You take a deep breath and hope that your lungs are okay. Then you rinse out the ice cream bowl (you didn't finish the ice cream), gather all your favorite orange-glazed Fiesta ware, and set them out on the back porch to ventilate. The next task is to open the encyclopedia to learn more about radon.

What is radon, anyway? Radon is a clear, odorless, natural gas that is produced through the decay of radium found in rocks and soil. It can seep into homes and buildings and into water systems, particularly in the northeastern United States. Radon is always a part of our atmosphere. However, when radon is trapped inside a home, the concentration can be considerably higher than when it is free in the atmosphere. If the radon level is greater than four "picocuries" (named after Madame Curie) per liter of air, people can become ill. And the orange Fiesta ware, you learned from the news account, releases up to twenty-eight picocuries per liter in a single room. The Environmental Protection Agency estimates that radon causes between seven thousand and thirty thousand lung cancer deaths per year in the United States alone (*Los Angeles Times*, 8 June 1994).

Fortunately, it's easy to determine how much radon might be in your house. Tests to measure radon levels cost only about $30. The Environmental Protection Agency has a voluntary program for identifying and reducing indoor radon pollution. The government is really *helping* here. Reducing radon levels in a building is simple. It usually means setting up a venting system to move air from the foundation and basements outside into the atmosphere. Good ventilation within a house also lowers radon levels.

But how about your grandmother's dishes? It seems that it's perfectly safe to collect and display them, as long they're in a well-ventilated room. It's just not such a good idea to serve food on them. You recall several years ago how the government issued warnings about certain glazes in Mexican pottery that contained lead. The stuff was beautiful to collect, but not safe to eat from. This seems like the same situation.

Your perspective begins to change. We're actually quite fortunate that the government notices and reports such potential problems. True, that orange Fiesta ware has been giving off radon for decades now, but modern science has become sophisticated enough to identify risks that we didn't know existed earlier. That might make things seem scarier — sometimes it feels like everything is dangerous — but it allows us to make wiser decisions about the risks we choose to accept.

You go into the kitchen, get out a newer dish (not as pretty as your grandmother's, but serviceable), and scoop some more ice cream. Yes, ice cream has fat in it, and fat is a risk to your arteries, but that is a risk worth taking tonight.

# LEAD-BASED PAINT: DANGER IN YOUR OWN HOME

If you buy a house or condominium in the United States, legally you have to sign an acknowledgement that you have received a certain warning letter. The letter shouts at you in capital letters: "WATCH OUT FOR LEAD-BASED PAINT POISONING!"

You cringe. Are you buying a death certificate for you and your children? The notice, issued by the U.S. Department of Housing and Urban Development, says that 3 out of 4 buildings built before 1978 have lead-based paint somewhere in or on the building. Exposure to this paint can poison children, especially those under age seven. Lead-based paint can damage the child's brain, nervous system, kidneys, vision, hearing, and coordination. A mother's exposure to lead-based paint can harm a fetus in the womb.

It seems that it's worth reading the fine print on this warning letter. For starters, everyone can get lead poisoning, including adults. It's simply worse for children because their bodies aren't yet fully formed and, of course, they're smaller. The same amount of lead exposure will cause proportionately more problems for them than for an adult. But you, too, can develop neurological problems — or worse — from ingesting lead from this paint.

Is it possible to get lead poisoning simply by living in a house that has some lead-based paint? What if the old paint is buried under a few layers of newer paint?

The problem with lead-based paint is that it doesn't just stay on the walls. For one thing, it chips. Opening a window can cause tiny bits of old paint, even paint a few layers down, to chip off. A toddler who is teething might chew on a windowpane and gnaw through to old paint. Soil next to buildings could have some chips of old lead paint, or lead paint dust, mixed in.

If you refinish old furniture, the paint that you remove could be lead-based, and paint chips and dust could end up in the cracks of your floorboards, to be breathed in by you and your loved ones.

So what do you do if you suspect that the paint in your charming old home might have lead in it? Should you scrape it off, then repaint? No, that's the worst thing you can do. Unfortunately the only way to get rid of lead-based paint safely is to pay a professional to do it — often for thousands of dollars. Qualified chemical and building firms, which you can locate by calling a local county health office, can test a home for lead-based paint. These expenses are worthwhile, especially if you have young children.

If you're worried about your child (or yourself), doctors can test the amount of lead in a person's blood. Many doctors recommend that a child be tested between the age of six months and one year, and at least annually after that if the child lives in an older house. The older the home, the worse the risk of lead-based poisoning.

Lead is a common substance, and by no means is it only found in old paint. It's also in colored newsprint and car batteries (especially the battery plate). So don't let your toddler chew on the Sunday comic pages—or the old car battery. Lead can enter your house through old pipes (which were made of lead and can contaminate the water) and through highly glazed pottery. You might have been advised to avoid buying pottery from Mexico. This pottery has been known to carry lead in the glaze. Eating from these plates can mean ingesting tiny bits of lead with each bite of food.

All this seems very depressing. Sometimes it feels as though we're not even safe in our own homes.

Fortunately, the risk of lead-based poisoning can be minimized to the point that it's negligible. Lead poisoning *is* something to be aware of, especially if you have children and live in an older home. However, if you live in an older house, you can have the place tested for lead-based paint and stripped of the risk. Houses built after 1979 carry little risk of lead-based paint, because this type of paint was banned in 1977. Neither you nor your child have to be the defenseless victims of your own home.

## ASBESTOS EVERYWHERE

The newspapers in Tanzania, a nation in East Africa, are filled with advertisements you'd never find in the United States: ads for the building material asbestos. Building companies in Tanzania promise that asbestos is safe, inexpensive, and the best insulation you'll find. Asbestos is fireproof, cheap, and strong, they assert. What more could you want?

In the United States, on the other hand, court calenders are filled with lawsuits for billions of dollars against asbestos companies. Asbestos has been proven to cause lung cancer and other lung diseases. The dangers of asbestos became known in the 1960s when hundreds of miners and industrial workers who had been exposed to asbestos developed deadly lung diseases. Asbestos was the very first material to be regulated by OSHA, the federal Occupational Safety and Health Administration.

The Environmental Protection Agency estimates that between three thousand and twelve thousand deaths from cancer each year in the United States are caused by asbestos exposure (*Grolier's Multimedia Encyclopedia*, 1993). The EPA and Congress have required asbestos use to be reduced by 94 percent by the late 1990s. The Third World, however, doesn't have this restriction, which is why cheap, efficient asbestos is used in those countries. Are the people in East Africa being sold a prescription for quick lung cancer? Or are we overreacting to asbestos in the United States? What *is* this deadly material asbestos, anyway?

The answers are no and yes to the first two questions. Asbestos does indeed cause cancer. The Environmental Protection Agency has ranked it as a Class A carcinogen. However, only certain types of asbestos are proven to cause cancer, and only if the asbestos is released into the atmosphere —

which it usually is not. Under normal circumstances it's kept tight and se-
cure within our walls and roofs. If we fear asbestos so much that we take drastic measures to avoid it entirely, we are overreacting. Used carefully for certain purposes, asbestos has advantages that actually outweigh its risks.

Let's look first at what asbestos really is, and then at how we've dealt with
the hazards associated with exposure to it. Asbestos comes from rock, which
is excavated from mines found all over the world, from Arizona to the Ap-
palachians, from Russia to California. The rock is hauled up from beneath
the earth's surface and crushed to release the fibers within. This fiber is then
spun or matted into insulation, fire-resistant safety tiles, and much more.

Asbestos can be found in your car's brake pads, probably in your roof and
flooring, in the cement in your patio, in the electrical insulation in your
walls . . . and maybe even in the heating insulation in your roof and walls.
More than half of all buildings that are over fifteen years old contain some
form of asbestos (*Los Angeles Times*, 10 February 1994). Asbestos really is
one of the world's best insulators. It's stable, strong, heat-resistant, fire-
resistant, and cheap. The advertisers in Tanzania are right.

Asbestos within home insulation and roofing is perfectly safe when it's kept
intact. It only gets dangerous when not kept intact. This can happen in a
typical home during renovations, or if the walls are crumbling (as in a very
old home) or are shaken apart, as in an earthquake. Asbestos inhalation was
a real threat in California, for example, during the January 1994 earthquake.
Health officials prevented many people from digging through their half-
collapsed homes or offices because asbestos fibers could have been released,
and people could breathe them in. Luckily for all of us, though, earthquakes are rare experiences.

Very low levels of asbestos are always floating around in the air, thanks to
the construction and demolition work usually going on somewhere nearby.
However, dozens of studies have shown that only those who work directly
with the material without protection for long periods of time are exposed to
health risks.

A scare in New York City shows how unnecessarily fearful we are of asbestos. In 1993, some chrysotile asbestos, the least toxic variety, was found
crumbling in several public schools. Although the schools had already been
inspected and deemed safe, parents went into a panic. Had the inspectors
lied? Newspapers carried the outrage on the front page; the evening news
jumped on the stories, too.

New York mayor David Dinkins responded to the upset parents and the
media with a promise that no schools would open until they all had been
re-inspected. Two weeks later, the reinspections were completed. But dur-

ing those two weeks, the one million kids who would have been in school were out on the streets — where they were in far more danger, as the *New York Times* (12 September 1994) sarcastically pointed out.

The costs of the reinspections in New York City ran over $120 million. Could that $120 million have been put to better use in the schools — for school lunches, maybe, or books, desks, computers, tutoring, you name it? That would be 120,000 computers . . . or 1.2 million books . . . or sixty million lunches. . . .

Later the *New York Times* (as quoted within the *Los Angeles Times*, 12 September 1994) quoted experts who pointed out that the whole scare was blown way out of proportion. Health and school officials were certain that the actual risk to a child was less than the statistical likelihood of being hit by lightning. As health experts and school officials said in the *Times* (12 September 1994), the reinspection was "based more on a need to reassure fearful parents than on any estimate of health risk."

Life as we know it has asbestos running through it. The only real risk from asbestos that most people face comes when homeowners, for example, might discover crumbling insulation (particularly on duct work) or fixtures. In that case it's best to hire a licensed asbestos contractor to see if the material contains asbestos. If you're nervous about your home, take advantage of several sources of free advice on asbestos inspection. Call your local chapters of the American Lung Association for their booklet "Asbestos in Your Home." Your County Health Department can also refer you to licensed asbestos inspectors.

Strangely enough, asbestos can be beautiful. Semiprecious gems, such as cat's-eye and tiger's-eye, can thank asbestos fibers buried within the stone for the lovely ripples and shadings that catch the light. In fact, you might even be wearing asbestos on your finger — and it won't hurt you there, just as it is unlikely to harm you in other places in your community.

# WILL VIDEO DISPLAY TERMINALS MAKE YOU "TERMINAL"?

**D**oes watching TV or working at the computer hurt a pregnant woman's developing child?

Lately some scientists have terrified us with a possible correlation between video display terminals, or VDTs, and an increased risk of miscarriage, birth defects, and (of course) cancer. You encounter a VDT every time you sit down at a computer or relax before the TV.

VDTs are potentially dangerous, some scientists say, because they generate electromagnetic fields (EMFs), the same electrical fields that come from power lines. EMFs are created by the flow of electrical charges in an alternating electrical current. The theory is that the vibrating electrical charges shake up the calcium ions in our cells, either killing the cells or preventing communication between cells. Although the frequencies on the VDT fields are much lower than those of power lines, they still might be strong enough to cause problems, especially if a woman spends many hours in front of the screen.

Or so the story goes.

Scientific studies have come to differing conclusions on the effects of VDTs on our health. The most important one, a seven-year study conducted by the National Institute for Occupational Safety and Health, found that women who work at VDTs do *not* have a higher rate of miscarriage. A British study arrived at a similar conclusion. Nevertheless, other researchers say that we should conduct more studies to *ensure* that VDTs don't hurt women's reproductive systems.

Some cities are playing it safe. San Francisco, for example, adopted a controversial law requiring businesses with more than fifteen people to provide

VDT "safeguards." These included chairs, lighting, and keyboards (to minimize wrist and back injury, eye strain, etc.) as well as VDT screens. On the other hand, similar proposed laws in other cities have failed because of their massive expense — all for the sake of uncertain research.

The VDT industry has given a lukewarm response to the controversy. They don't seem terribly worried. Some computer makers, but not all, sell terminals with shields that reduce some low-level EMFs. Sweden and Denmark, which strictly regulate workplace conditions, lead the field in these innovations.

Realistically, VDTs are just one of many sources of everyday exposure to electromagnetic fields, including TVs, hair dryers, blenders, electric blankets, power tools, anything that has an alternating electrical current. Are we going to do away with our computers and toasters because we're worried about the potential risks of EMFs? There is no research on *which* electrical devices, and how *much* of those devices, cause *which* types of diseases — if any at all.

Electricity, and the thousands of inventions it spawned, have saved thousands of lives. Electricity also has improved the quality of our lives immeasurably. Which would you rather do: turn off all the lights (are you reading by electrical light right now?), never blow-dry your hair in the morning, not run the dishwasher, never fax anything again or use the computer, make no more margaritas in the blender, let your dinner thaw for hours instead of zapping it in the microwave, never toast your bread, use a manual instead of an electric lawnmower, throw away your stereo . . . *or* risk the minuscule, undocumented possibility of cancer. Take your choice.

# BIOTECHNOLOGY FOR BREAKFAST: SUPER-COW OR COW VILLAIN?

The latest biotechnology has made it to your breakfast table. Much of the milk sold today has been produced using "bovine growth hormone," or BGH. What exactly is BGH, and why are health-food stores carrying "organic" milk labeled "no growth hormones"? Should we be worried about BGH?

Biotechnology is the newest kid on the block in our many attempts to increase food production. Biotechnology works by cloning genes to make a "better" tomato, for example, or a cow that produces more milk. Cows injected with synthetic bovine growth hormone created in a laboratory increase their milk production by 10 to 25 percent (*Tufts University Diet & Nutrition Letter*, April 1994). But is the milk that comes from these cows any different than other milk? Isn't this process "unnatural" in some way?

Cows treated with genetically created bovine growth hormone do tend to have a slightly higher incidence of mastitis, a swelling of the udder. Farmers frequently treat this problem with antibiotics, which potentially could end up in a cow's milk.

The U.S. Congress shared these concerns. The Food and Drug Administration approved BGH in late 1993, but Congress prevented BGH from being sold for ninety days. Congress wanted to study the impact of BGH on "human safety, animal health and well-being, economic change, ethics, farm structure and incomes, the environment, investment in biotechnology, rural social life, and other issues," according to the Clinton administration.

Over the ninety days, various federal agencies reviewed the scientific evidence for BGH and wrote reports . . . and more reports . . . and more reports. There are now over fifteen hundred studies, books, papers, and surveys on BGH, more than on any other animal drug.

Congress finally allowed the sale of BGH to begin because they found "no evidence" that BGH "poses a health threat to humans or animals." Congress's report noted that the hormone has also been found safe by many other scientific bodies in the United States, including the National Institutes for Health and the Office of Technology Assessment, as well as the drug regulatory agencies of Canada, the United Kingdom, and the European Union.

The government has become so sure about the safety of BGH that milk sellers aren't required to label milk that came from cows injected with BGH, since, the FDA says, the milk is indistinguishable from non-BGH milk. Bovine–growth-hormone milk is "natural" because cows produce this hormone naturally. And bovine growth hormone is destroyed during pasteurization anyway.

So as we pour milk over our cereal in the morning, should we worry? No. In fact, bovine growth hormone is *good* for us and our environment. We're so conditioned to crying "cancer!" to any sort of fiddling with foods — whether by pesticide, preservative, or biotechnology — that we often ignore the benefits of new technology. First of all, milk farmers can receive more milk from fewer cows. Second, because we will need fewer dairy cows, we'll need less grain and grazing lands to feed the cows. This means less fertilizer needed to grow grain, and thus less fertilizer run off into the groundwater. We'll have more open land available because we need smaller pastures.

Of course, the biggest beneficiaries of bovine growth hormone may be the companies who make and sell it to dairy farmers. Nevertheless, adding up the pros and cons, it seems that even if BGH carried a minuscule health risk, the environmental gains might actually outweigh the risk. If a product produces far greater benefit than harm, we can hardly call it risky.

So why do health food stores sell milk labeled "no bovine growth hormones"? It could be because some people are scared of any new technology, even when it's proven safe. Also, some people don't trust agencies such as the Food and Drug Administration, or even Congress, for political reasons and don't believe their reassurances of safety. And some people have simply bought into the "buy natural" campaign at any cost. Milk marketed as "natural" is quite costly, but actually most agree that it is indistinguishable from the rest of the milk on the supermarket shelves.

# URBAN/SUBURBAN
# SURVIVAL

# THE SAFE MEAN STREETS

**M**ad gunmen shooting innocent victims as they commute home from work on a train. Drive-by shootings. Gang murders. Car and home break-ins. Robberies around the corner. These days people are more worried about crime than ever before.

We're putting our money where our fear is. By some estimates, Americans have spent $50 billion, or almost $200 for every man, woman, and child in the country, on security devices ranging from sophisticated home alarm systems, to artificial dogs that bark when they sense movement, to full-fledged auto-security systems, to car steering-wheel locks.

Are we more threatened than ever? Not according to the Justice Department. The Department's Bureau of Justice Statistics has been compiling crime reports for more than twenty years. It reported in 1993 that the overall number of crime victimizations had *dropped* 6 percent since 1973.

Still, crime rates *are* high. In 1993, 1 in 4 U.S. households had at least one family member who was a crime victim. But did you know that the percentage was actually far *higher* twenty years ago? In 1975, the Justice Department reported that 1 in 3 households was victimized by crime.

The encouraging statistics go on. In 1994, nonviolent and violent crimes reported to the police dropped for the third year in a row. And in the same year big cities became *safer*, not more dangerous. Urban areas with populations over one million saw a 6 percent drop in reported crime (*Outlook*, 22 May 1995).

White households have done particularly well. In 1992, the Justice Department reported that the percentage of white households experiencing crimes was at its lowest level ever. African-Americans have not experienced additional crime since 1989, although crime rates are still higher than average in these communities. The proportion of African-American households suffering from crime has stayed about the same for the past five years.

But you'd never know any of these facts from the headlines, local television news reports, and all those stump speeches we hear as politicians campaign. All of the focus is on the most dramatic and violent crimes, especially crimes involving increasingly powerful weapons, even though they represent only a small proportion of overall crime.

No wonder our concern about crime has been skyrocketing, even though statistics point the other way. In early 1994, more than 40 percent of Americans ranked crime as the country's most important problem. That's a huge increase from just three years earlier, when only a tiny percentage of the population cited crime as an important national problem.

In this section, we'll look at crime in cars, at home, and in the office. We'll review the variety of self-defense devices on the market. How safe are you? How safe are you with a can of Mace or an auto-security system? Read on.

## YOUR HOME IS YOUR FORTRESS

For Billy and Fyrn Davis, their home *was* a fortress. The couple, who lived in a two-story home in the quiet Los Angeles suburb of Pico Rivera, were so worried about crime that they put bars on their windows. That wasn't so unusual, but for the Davises, it was just the beginning. They also installed video monitors, infrared alarms, and five-hundred-watt spotlights in the yard. They built a spike and razor-wire fence.

The media seized on Billy and Fyrn Davis as a symbol of the fear of crime and violence that has gripped us. But did all their precautions save the Davises? Unfortunately not. In fact, in this case they caused more harm than good.

The day after Billy lost his battle against illness in a hospital, a report of fire sent fire fighters rushing to Fyrn Davis's house. But the extra locks delayed them entering for half an hour. When the fire fighters finally burst through the front door, they found Fyrn Davis's charred corpse in the living room. She couldn't get out, and they couldn't get in.

Protecting yourself from the world's dangers can also mean *preventing* yourself from accessing the many safeguards and services our society has created.

"People aren't even safe in their homes anymore." How often have you heard that angry remark? People all over feel that their last refuge, the one place where they thought they could escape crime and the problems of modern life, is no longer a safe haven. Everyone knows someone whose home has been broken into. Stories about innocent people being murdered in their homes abound.

Are we, in fact, more threatened than ever before, even in our homes? No.

Since 1973, the Justice Department has documented declines in many crimes. The steepest drops have come in household burglary and theft, which fell 6 percent in 1993 alone. That's even the case if you live in a big house in a prosperous neighborhood, which some people think would make you a target for burglars. But in fact, federal statistics show just the opposite: as household income rises, burglary rates fall.

One of the biggest factors determining how safe you are at home is where you live. In 1992, murder rates were 81 percent lower in the suburbs than in big cities. Robbery rates were almost 90 percent lower in the suburbs than in big cities. And rates of rape were 56 percent lower (*Los Angeles Times*, 7 July 1994).

This doesn't mean everyone is less likely to be a crime victim. If you're a young minority male living in a central city, for example, your chances of being victimized are higher than ever: 1 in 6.

But wherever you live, you can do a lot to make yourself less likely to be victimized in your home. Police say that more than seven million residential burglaries occur each year (*Los Angeles Times*, 21 May 1994). That is a frightening statistic. But even more frightening is how little residents do to prevent themselves from joining these statistics — and without spending thousands on expensive alarm systems. Of those seven million burglaries, *nearly half* occur without force. That means the criminals entered through unlocked doors and windows. So the first, and one of the most effective, steps you can take to avoid crime at home is to take the simple and obvious step of being sure that you keep your doors and windows locked. There are other easy ways to reduce your chances of becoming a victim. Never leave a house key under a doormat, in a flower pot, or on the ledge of a door. These may be obvious places to hide a key, but they are equally obvious to someone trying to sneak into your home. And be careful about opening the door to strangers. Insist that unexpected visitors identify themselves and explain why they are there.

Another strategy police endorse is starting or joining a neighborhood watch program. These exist in virtually every community in the country, and are a good way to get to know your neighbors. This builds bonds among people with a common interest in preventing crime and makes it all the more obvious when strangers are hanging around.

Keep this information and these statistics in mind the next time you see one of those dramatic stories on the local television news about the latest person who suffered a vicious attack in their home. It does happen, but it's not nearly so common as the media lead you to believe. And you can do a lot to make yourself safe by carefully choosing where you live, keeping your doors and windows locked, and, as always, by staying alert.

# ROAD WARRIORS

As you finish up the last few lines of a report your boss wants in the morning, you glance up at the clock on your office wall and notice . . . you're late. It's already 7:45 P.M., and you're supposed to be meeting a business friend at a new restaurant on the other side of town in fifteen minutes. You'll never make it. You gather up the fancy brochures you need and rush into the parking garage — which is dark and nearly empty.

Not many people seem to work as late as you do. The garage feels a bit eerie with so few cars. You hurry across the concrete floor toward your reliable old clunker, fumble with the keys, get in, and begin unlocking your Club. It's great to have one of these steel steering-wheel locks, you think. After all, you've seen the ads with the cop in his fancy blue uniform telling you how many cars are stolen each year, even in office-building parking lots. And it's cheaper than an expensive alarm system — which goes off so frequently in parking structures anyway that you wonder how effective they really are. But as you swivel your head to check for suspicious-looking strangers, you wish you didn't have to waste the extra few minutes unlocking the antitheft device.

There, it's open. You pull out of the garage and onto the street. So far, so good.

You're halfway to the restaurant, located in an unfamiliar part of town, when you remember that you're out of cash. A few blocks later, you see a bank with a well-lighted automated teller machine, and pull into the driveway. But as you wait for the machine to spit out the crisp green bills, you begin to get nervous. Your recall all those stories about people being robbed, even killed, at ATMs. You quickly stuff the wad of twenty-dollar bills into your pocket and pull out onto the street.

Dinner is great. Your business friend likes your ideas and, besides, you like each other. You agree to have these get-togethers more often. As you head for your car, you notice that it's almost midnight, a lot later than you expected. You were having fun, weren't you? But at this hour, you don't feel comfortable driving back the way you came. The neighborhood didn't look very appealing.

Instead, you decide to head home on the freeway. It's longer, but at least you won't be stuck at stoplights at dark intersections. Once you're on the free-way, a car pulls up behind you, a bit too close. Why don't they just pass, you wonder. Then they do. The beat-up old Chevy is packed with four or five young guys, who look over and laugh as they pull ahead of you. Then the Chevy pulls into your lane, slows down, speeds up, slows down again. Now what? You turn up the radio, and mentally calculate how much farther until you reach your exit. Fifteen minutes.

As you stare straight ahead, the guys in the Chevy pull into the next lane and slow down until they're right beside you. One of the guys points his index finger at you, and instinctively, you duck. For a second, you thought it was a gun. This isn't Los Angeles, but freeway shootings can happen anywhere, can't they? You try to ignore the young toughs, checking your rearview mir-ror for other cars on the freeway. The game continues for a few more min-utes — or is it hours? — until the teenagers get bored, and pull off at an exit you've never heard of. When they're gone, you notice that your heart is pounding. It's not safe anywhere anymore, is it? Not even in your car.

All this fear of crime on the freeway, of car theft, and of being robbed in a parking lot has shaped American consumers. For example, they have bought more than 14 million Clubs — the antitheft device that locks steering wheels — since they went on the market in 1986, and the trend continues. Analysts expect consumers to increase their spending on auto protection de-vices by 30 to 50 percent during the next decade (*Los Angeles Times*, 17 De-cember 1994).

But will products such as the Club keep your car from being stolen? Prob-ably not, according to criminologist Marcus Felson. Felson doesn't mince words. Most security devices, he says, are "a waste of money." Although *Con-sumer Reports* magazine says the Club is a deterrent to theft, the magazine added that any determined thief could make quick work of it. The maga-zine's testers noted that "we could easily slice through the steering wheel and slip the lock off like a ring from a finger."

Fortunately, given that such devices as the Club aren't 100 percent ef-fective, your chances of having your car stolen aren't great anyway — unless you belong to a high-risk group. According to the Highway Loss Data Institute, car theft is highest in New York City, and the Mercedes SL convertible and other high-end sports cars are car thieves' favorite targets. Large cars are less likely to be stolen. In 1993, for example, auto thefts declined by 4 percent. What can be effective in preventing car theft are the factory-installed antitheft devices that disconnect a car's electrical system or start sirens when a window is broken or a door forced open.

But don't spend too much money on security, unless you're in one of those high-risk groups. Many experts say that spending money on security systems, even sophisticated ones, isn't the answer.

How about carjacking? This "new" crime has made headlines across the nation, even making its way into presidential and congressional crime bills as a truly heinous crime worthy of at least fifteen years in prison. The *Chicago Tribune* reported in June 1995 that, ironically, carjacking is "a crime driven by improved anti-theft technology and alarm systems on parked cars." If the thieves can't get into parked cars, they'll try while you're driving.

Carjacking actually isn't nearly as common as the headlines would lead us to believe. According to a 1995 Justice Department report, a motorist's risk of being carjacked is 1 in 5,000, or the same risk as dying in a traffic accident. That means that only 2 in every 10,000 Americans are victims of a carjacking attempt each year. This is compared to 5 in 5,000 who are victims of attempted rape, or 25 out of 5,000 who die of heart disease. Of course, no one wants to be any of these statistics, but they can help us put the carjacking risk in perspective.

There were 177,500 carjackings attempted from 1987 to 1992, according to the Bureau of Justice Statistics. Of these, 60 percent involved handguns, and weapons in general were used in 80 percent of the cases. Black motorists were twice as likely as whites to be victims, and men are three times more likely than women to be victims. Most important of all, only 4 percent of carjacking victims are seriously injured, stabbed, or shot. Only 52 percent of carjackings are successful. Although the 1994 carjacking murder of two Japanese students in Los Angeles made international news, it was truly an exception to the typical carjacking scenario.

How can you protect yourself against carjacking, and auto theft in general? The best way to keep from becoming a victim in your car is to take a few simple precautions: park in a well-lighted spot, close all your windows (professional thieves need only a tiny amount of open space to open your car), lock your doors, have your keys ready and hold them firmly in your fist, and get a friend to accompany you or ask to be escorted when you need to go into a dark parking lot. Also, check in and around your car to be sure that there is no one lurking nearby or hidden in the backseat. And, if you suspect that someone might be following you, don't lead them to your house. Instead, head for the nearest police station, or at least to a well-lighted commercial place with plenty of activity around. Keep your doors locked, even in "safe" areas, and stay alert at lonely or dark intersections.

So the next time you consider investing money in auto security devices . . . think again. Common sense may do a lot more to protect you, for a lot less, than any security system you could buy. And the next time you worry whether to go out at night in your car, fearing carjacking, consider the statistics about this actual risk — and the many ways you can reduce your risk by applying common sense.

# A CALL TO ARMS

**W**e feel more and more threatened by crime. Opinion polls in the United States show that the public ranks crime as the country's No. 1 problem. This fear is often not related to how likely someone is to actually be a *victim* of crime. White women, for example, tend to express the greatest fear of crime. Ironically, they are also the least likely to be crime victims.

An elderly white woman's chances of being the victim of violent crime in any year are less than one-fourth of 1 percent. This age group is the *least* likely to be touched by crime. Yet our mothers and grandmothers are often so frightened that they dare not go out at night.

Three criminologists who extensively studied crime and the perception of crime wrote a book in 1993 entitled *The Mythology of Crime and Criminal Justice*. The three researchers, Victor E. Kappeler, Gary W. Potter, and Mark Blumberg, concluded that people's understanding of crime is obscured by political and commercial myths. Hard facts are frequently manipulated. The book concludes that we are filled with *unnecessary fear* that sometimes makes us not more, but *less*, safe. And the power of modern communication gives these distortions all the more power.

The media are the main influence on public perception of the threat of crime. One recent poll found that 72 percent of small town residents and 69 percent of suburban residents say their feelings about crime are evoked most by what the media tell them. A third of those surveyed reported that they became more fearful of crime because of specific incidents reported in the press (*Los Angeles Times*, 13 February 1994). This comes without regard to their actual risk of being a crime victim.

The result is that millions of people have lost faith in the ability of the police and the criminal justice system to protect them. So they've decided to take steps to protect themselves. One in 4 Americans now arms himself or herself outside the home.

In the 1990s, fear sells. Advertisers have picked up on all the media hype about crime and now hawk dozens of devices that are supposed to protect your body from assault and your property from theft. In 1993 alone, Americans spent more than $400 million on safety equipment and services.

Guns are the most notorious items Americans have been buying to protect themselves. Even former first lady Nancy Reagan kept a small silver pistol near her bed. Americans now own millions of handguns. But most law enforcement studies have found that owning a gun makes you more vulnerable to being shot, not less.

Many people who don't like the idea of carrying a gun have taken up other forms of self-defense. Mace. Pepper spray. Stun guns. Noise alarms. Smell repellents, and more. But do they work? A recent investigation by the *Los Angeles Times* (8 July 1994) yielded decidedly mixed results.

Take Mace, for example. Mace is the brand name for a kind of tear gas that inflames the eyes, nose, and throat. Getting sprayed with Mace is painful, and experts say it *will* deter many assailants. But not all. A former member of the California Highway Patrol, Warren Clark, told the *Los Angeles Times* (8 July 1994), "If you handled a garden-variety combatant, it would work," but "If you handled someone highly intoxicated with cocaine, PCP or alcohol, you'd get them angry and probably be in for a pretty good fight."

Stun guns are another option. These "guns" are equipped with metal prongs that deliver an electric shock when applied to someone. But you have to get close enough to an attacker to touch his or her skin with the prongs. Someone wearing heavy clothing may not be affected. And if you don't surprise an assailant, he or she may disarm you. In that case, you might end up being a double victim.

Noise alarms are most commonly found on cars, though many personal safety versions exist, too. These are often very small, and are designed to attract attention and frighten away an assailant. But crime experts agree they have limited effectiveness. Says Los Angeles Police Department crime specialist Lt. Chris West, "If you're in a mall parking lot where they could hear and come to your aid, it's a great system. But if you're in a subterranean garage at 9:00 or 10:00 at night all by yourself, who's going to hear you?" The detective adds, "How much attention do you pay to car alarms?"

It's so easy to get caught up in the hysteria over crime that it becomes difficult to keep perspective. Here are a few government figures that might surprise you. Each year, your chances of injuring yourself in some kind of accident — any kind — are more than 1 in 5. Your chances of being injured by someone out to do you harm are a little over 1 in 100. That means, on average, you'd have to live to be almost a hundred years old before being injured in a crime.

Before you let the paranoia of life in the modern world assail you, consider carefully what *really* deters crime. Guns, Mace, and noise alarms might help. But the best method may not be any of these products touted so heavily in advertisements and the press. In fact, some experts say steering clear of crime has more to do with something as simple as how you look, rather than how you're armed. You may avoid more trouble simply by staying alert and at least *appearing* confident. "The robber typically avoids people who are alert," says University of Southern California criminology specialist Marcus Felson.

There are some simple ways to make it clear to potential assailants that you are paying attention. Police suggest obviously looking at people around you, staying in well-lighted places, walking close to the curb, walking confidently and without hesitation, and making eye contact with other people on the street. A few more tips: Hold your purse or other personal belongings securely near your body, have your keys ready before you reach your car, and do not carry large amounts of cash. You might want to consider direct deposit for your pay or social security checks. And if you are held up, police routinely advise victims to give robbers what they ask for. That won't guarantee your physical safety, but it is less likely to provoke an assailant to attack you violently. After all, no material possession is more important than your life.

So the next time you think about loading yourself up with dangerous new toys, think again. You may do more to protect yourself by paying attention and looking self-assured. And that's good advice whether or not you're worried about becoming a victim of crime.

# WORK CAN KILL YOU: DEATH ON THE JOB

The images remain etched in our minds: a huge office building, ripped open from top to bottom, the bodies of more than a hundred innocent people buried under the rubble. Within days after the bombing of the main federal office building in downtown Oklahoma City in May 1995, employers all over the country began taking action — hiring extra security guards, inspecting bags and briefcases, and (in many government office buildings) erecting concrete barriers to keep terrorists and criminals from parking potential car bombs close to buildings.

It's happening everywhere, isn't it? We hear about angry and deranged postal workers who shoot at their fellow employees, mad loners who take out their unhappiness on customers and employees at fast-food restaurants, and drug-crazed patients assaulting doctors and nurses. Almost every month, we see a new headline or another TV news story about seemingly senseless or random violence perpetrated against employees just trying to do their jobs and bring home their paychecks.

The U.S. Department of Justice reported in 1994 that fully 1 in 6 violent crimes occurs in the workplace — or 1 million violent crimes each year. Of these, about 10 percent involve offenders with handguns. Seven percent of the nation's rapes, 8 percent of robberies, and 16 percent of assaults occur on the job. Most of these assaults come from strangers, not co-workers. Federal employees suffer the brunt of this workplace violence: although they make up only 18 percent of the work force, they experience 30 percent of the workplace violence. This may be because these employees are more exposed to the public — often a disgruntled public. And as in the Oklahoma City bombing, people might take out their frustrations with government on the government's hapless employees.

Both government and private employers are responding to these threats. Some cautiously check prospective employees' backgrounds to see if they have criminal records. Others administer psychological tests, even though the results of these tests often are inconclusive, at best. Some managers are said to wear bulletproof vests when they fire workers. Workers who have hiring responsibility are being trained to look for signs of stress in applicants. Employers also are trying to find ways to reduce the strain of high-stress jobs.

Politicians, who never want to be behind a trend, have begun introducing legislation to try to reduce workplace violence. In 1993, the Labor Department conducted its first-ever serious study on the subject and reported that 1,004 people were victims of work-related homicides in 1992. In fact, for women, homicide was the top cause of work fatalities. The Federal Occupational Safety and Health Administration is also trying to devise strategies to cut down on violence at work. A whole new field comprised of psychologists and management consultants has evolved to counsel frightened employees and to tell employers what precautions they should take.

Many companies and commercial establishments have installed buzzers or other security devices that encourage employees to observe or speak with people trying to enter. The managers of skyscrapers in major cities often have security offices that require all people entering without employee identification to register, list the person being visited, have that person approve the visitor's entry, and then wear a visitor's badge visibly at all times.

And when was the last time you saw your "mug" on a video monitor — at a convenience store, a gas station, a bank, a retail store . . . and the list goes on? Probably within the past week. Video surveillance is meant to protect employees and businesses from violence and theft. Post offices and banks in high-risk areas often have bulletproof shields between workers and customers (sad but true). Some companies have drafted safety and security regulations, and employees are required to attend personal security seminars. Other workplaces have taken care to light parking areas thoroughly; others provide escort services if needed.

Remember, too, the adage "safety in numbers." A solitary worker in an office at night should take care to lock the doors and alert Security that he or she is working alone. But for the rest of us, working in offices or factories with many other people around, we can take comfort in "numbers."

Workplace violence is a symptom of our times. In the 1990s, people all over are wondering whether they'll make it home after they leave for work in the morning. But how serious is this threat? How likely are you to be the victim of violent crime on the job?

After taking a good hard look at the statistics, what can you conclude about workplace violence that will help put the dangers in perspective? Certainly, some jobs do carry risks. Examples are working as an armored car driver, a bank teller in a crime-ridden inner city, or a door-to-door salesperson, at a convenience or liquor store, or as a cab driver. But in most jobs, you're very unlikely to be hurt. Think of the millions of people who go to work each day. Each year we complete billions of workdays. How many incidents of workplace violence do you hear about? Not many.

News about workplace violence has only just begun to hit the radio airwaves, television stations, and newspaper stands. Although this news scares us, the fact that we're hearing about it is good: we're aware of the issue, and many companies and organizations are taking steps to *prevent* workplace violence before it increases.

# FEAR OF FLYING

The jumbo jet is about to taxi down to the runway. You're breaking out into a cold sweat. There was a plane crash last week, killing all 158 people on board. When you said good-bye to your wife at the airport, you wondered if you'd ever see her again. But you didn't say anything. She'd just worry. Airplanes are supposed to be safe, right? Safer than driving. That's what you've heard.

The plane turns a corner on the runway. Red and white lights are flashing outside the tiny window. God, you hope the pilot knows what he's doing. Over the intercom, he tells the passengers what the weather's like at thirty thousand feet. You wish he'd shut up and pay attention to the runway. The flight attendants have finished playing the safety video, and they are strapped into their safety seats. You studiously watched the video, even though you've seen dozens of times how oxygen masks fall from the over-head compartment, how the seat cushion converts to a flotation device, how the exit doors open. . . .

You're sitting over the wing and next to the exit door because they're the safest places on an airplane, you've heard — except on DC-10s, a couple of which cracked down the middle ten years ago or so, you recall. But this isn't a DC-10. Nor is it one of those commuter planes that crash more often than big jets. In fact, even though it's a lot less convenient, you're taking this jumbo jet flight rather than the little commuter plane that would have been less expensive. The danger here is wind shear, poor air traffic control, pilot error — all of which lead to crashes and fire. You check the seat pocket in front of you, where you've stowed your smoke hood. It was expensive — $70 — but worth it. Most people in plane crashes die from smoke inhalation, not the impact of the crash. You won't be one of them. . . . And right about now that flight insurance you bought is looking like a great deal.

Have you ever experienced such fear of flying? Most of us have, even though we still take airplane flights. How can we avoid such fear when newspapers and television news broadcast gory photographs of plane crashes? "How Safe Is This Flight?" demands a *Newsweek* (24 April 1995) magazine cover story. The story's subtitle warns, "Hundreds of Americans died in commercial-airplane crashes in 1994. . . . And as air travel grows, the risks can only increase."

Are these fears grounded? Is it true that as air travel grows, the risks will increase? Is the unusually high number of crashes in the past couple of years a sign that airplanes are a dangerous way to travel? Are the hundreds of people who have a "fear of flying" justified in their fears?

*Newsweek*, along with dozens of other magazines, newspapers, and television programs, tells us in minute detail about the tragedies of air crashes: "The cabin shattered into a gruesome tangle of metal, bags and bodies — including that of a 9-month-old baby ripped from her mother's arms" (24 April 1995). Pictures of crash scenes are splashed across the front pages of newspapers. When a large airplane crash occurs, it leads the news. The entire world is riveted on the tragedy. The media talk of little else.

The ValuJet crash on 11 May 1996 commanded headlines for two months. And it truly was a tragedy—all 110 people on board were killed. However, even this tragedy has had the positive effect of ensuring even more stringent standards of safety. Although the investigation has indicated human error as the likeliest cause of this crash—unsafe oxygen containers were loaded on the airplane—this disaster has helped to point out other areas where safety officials can now focus more effectively. Further, the FAA is now paying closer attention to the smaller airlines and the charter industry. And also, Congress is considering overhauling the Federal Aviation Administration, making it even more effective in preventing disasters like the ValuJet crash in the Florida Everglades.

And as if the looming threat of human error or unstable weather weren't already making you feel ill at ease with air travel, there still exists the off chance that some unhappy political faction might seize this opportunity to right their political wrongs through the drastic means of terrorism. And to make matters worse, the media are quick to sound the alarmist sirens prior to determining what may not have actually occurred.

There is no better example of this than with the recent disaster of TWA flight 800 on 17 July 1996. The media hastily created an atmosphere of con-

trolled hysteria before the actual cause of the disaster had even been established. Newspaper and television reporters quickly gathered what little they
knew of the tragedy and instantly leapt to create an atmosphere of frenzy
and fear. These reports only helped to expose our already-vulnerable suspi-
cions of the flying industry. And for what? Improved ratings?

It is difficult enough to filter through the actual facts without having a
litany of nonscientific information reported based strictly on speculation and
hearsay. And while at the time of this publication the cause of this horrible
disaster has yet to be determined, we can receive some comfort from the fact
that Bill Clinton has signed a new airline safety and security measure that
will tighten regulations on airlines and will help further reduce any threat
to our well-being and personal safety. And while we may be upset with the
media for creating an atmosphere of panic and suspicion, they are at least
indirectly responsible for helping prompt the government to heed our concerns and take a step forward toward securing the airways we travel. But is
the heightened security really necessary? Will the public tolerate increased
delays at airport check-ins, and increased costs of travel to pay for these security measures? Only time will tell.

As you stare at those crash site pictures, worrying about your next flight,
wondering if you should *drive* across the country instead, even though the
trip would take five days instead of five hours, stop for a moment. Step back
from the horrifying pictures and frightening headlines. Ask yourself *why* the
latest airline crash received so much attention.

*Because it's so rare.* This is the *good news* hidden in the very nature of
media coverage on airplane crashes and the attention we pay to it. The media
focus so much on plane crashes because they're infrequent. Each day, U.S.
airlines make 30,000 flights with more than 1.5 million passengers on board
(*Newsweek*, 24 April 1995). Let's take a hypothetical example. Even if there
are five major crashes a year, killing 200 people each, that's 5 out of almost
11 *million* flights that year and 1,000 out of over 547 *billion* passengers who
took flights that year. Thus the chances of dying in a plane crash are about
the same as being hit by lightning (*Los Angeles Times*, 23 June 1996).

It's true that the media also pay attention to airplane crashes because
they're catastrophic, often killing many people at once. Airplane crashes are
horrible and shouldn't be trivialized. However, in terms of sheer numbers
of fatalities, air travel is far, far safer than many other "risks" we face in modern society.

Here's another way of slicing the statistics. Arnold Barnett of the Massachusetts Institute of Technology has reviewed the numbers of flights, pas-

sengers, and airline crashes. Until 1994, the U.S. domestic airline industry was the safest in the world. The 1994 accidents brought down those statistics. Nevertheless, the "death risk" of flying on jets (both domestic and international) from 1985 to 1994, as reported by *Newsweek* (24 April 1995), ranges from "zero" (for 8 out of 16 airlines reviewed) to 1 in 100 million (2 out of the 16) to 1 in 1 million. What does this mean? You would have to take, on average, from 1 million to 100 million flights before the plane would crash. The likelihood of crashing is extremely small. As *Newsweek* points out, the risk of drowning in the bathtub is ten times higher.

In fact, FAA administrator David Hinson points out that the accident rate in airlines has *dropped* 85 percent since the 1960s, even while the number of flights has *doubled.*

By the way, turbulence while flying isn't anything to be scared about. It's only dangerous if the plane is taking off or landing. Nor is lightning dangerous while you're flying. If lightning hits a plane, you might hear an explosion and see a flash of light, and then perhaps see a burn mark on the side of the plane. But that's it.

The frightened man at the opening of this chapter is right when he thinks that the risk is somewhat greater with U.S. commuter planes (the smaller prop or turboprop planes that make little "hops" between cities). The risk there ranges from zero to 1 in 1 million (this worst statistic comes from Alaska, where weather conditions can be severe) (*Newsweek,* 24 April 1995).

Well — are you convinced that it's safe to fly? Maybe. But the next time you're strapped into your seat and accelerating down a runway, will you be nervous *anyway* — in spite of all the reassuring statistics?

Probably. We're vulnerable hurling through space at up to five hundred miles per hour, thirty-five thousand feet above the earth, encased in a metal tube with wings. We are forced to trust the pilots, the air traffic controllers, the pilots of other planes in the sky around us, and the many manufacturers of the plane and its thousands of parts. We do not have control of our destinies or our safety. We have placed our lives in someone else's hands. That's scary no matter how objectively "safe" the situation might be.

The next time you take off in an airplane, searching the sky nervously for thunderclouds, think about this silver lining. The extensive media coverage of any airplane accident has led to higher scrutiny on air transportation safety. When the media make a fuss about airline safety, government policy makers are forced to listen and act. U.S. Department of Transportation secretary Federico Pena is taking dramatic steps to improve air transportation safety. The inspector general of the U.S. Department of Transportation is conducting dozens of prosecutions against the FAA to ensure greater safety. Rather than letting our fears drive us toward danger (such as driving a car across the country rather than flying), we can use the fear to make changes in the system to make it even safer.

# OUR
## ENVIRONMENT

# THE GREEN MONSTER

It lurks in your television set and in the front section of your newspaper. It jumps out of your car radio as you drive home. It lives in your mailbox during political campaigns.

What is it? The environmental monster — which has two faces. One side, viewed by the environmentalists, carries an expression of continual doom. The world is going to heat up and be swallowed by its oceans; in fifty years we won't be able to breathe our own air; all water is polluted; we're going to blow ourselves up; we've killed our Mother Earth. . . . This face of the monster has a dark scowl, an angry brow, a big mouth, the trail of a dried tear on a cheek, and an intelligent, calculating glint in the eyes. This face of the monster terrifies us.

The other face of the green monster is favored by the capitalists, industrialists, and consumers. It's smiling and affable, ready to offer itself up like a servant. Maybe the smile is a bit too false and the teeth too white, like the grin of a salesman about to clinch an advantageous deal. This side of the face looks confident that the world will never die. We will all live and become rich. It is the face of greed, ready to ravage the countryside for a quick buck. There's enough of everything to go around. This optimistic attitude is reassuring, true enough; but we wonder if it's deceptive. Are we lying to ourselves? Are we poisoning our earth?

No matter which way you look at it, the environmental monster pops up everywhere these days. We continually hear about the environmental debate. Is the ozone layer thinning? — or is that just a myth — or is the issue so complicated that no easy answer is possible? Is our groundwater polluted, or is that just a sales pitch created by the springwater companies and the environmentalists? Is the government right in allowing timber companies to cut trees on public lands, or are they permitting the destruction of one of our most important natural resources for the sake of a few jobs and huge corporate profits? Which is right?

Can some of the environmentalists' assertions be true and others false? Which are hyperbole, which understatement? What should we do about the environmental problems that *are* serious? Or, as environment reporter Gregg Easterbrook points out in his 1995 book *A Moment on the Earth: The Coming Age of Environmental Optimism,* perhaps we've done such a good job protecting our environment since the first Earth Day twenty-five years ago (thanks to the environmentalists' outcries) that we can ease up a bit.

This section takes aim at the green monster. We'll delve into several of the scariest caves inhabited by this monster and shine a flashlight on the walls. Maybe the monster isn't as scary as it seems. Maybe the world isn't coming to an end, at least not quite yet.

# THE GREENHOUSE EFFECT: A STORY OF HOT AIR?

I t's too darn hot," Ella Fitzgerald crooned. And she might not have seen the worst of it by a long shot, according to many scientists.

Thanks to greater carbon dioxide emissions, mostly from cars and factories, we've turned up the atmospheric heat. The earth is cooking — some might say "stewing in its own juices." The alleged result? Farmlands will dry up. Plants and animals will die. Polar ice caps will melt, flooding coastal cities around the world. All of this will come as a result of the "greenhouse effect," a process by which carbon dioxide released into the air traps heat and keeps it in our atmosphere.

Are we ruining our planet? The former head of the Environmental Protection Agency, William Reilly, sees the greenhouse effect as the most serious environmental problem facing the United States. In *Earth in the Balance: Ecology and the Human Spirit* (1992), Vice President Al Gore called the greenhouse effect an "ecological crisis without precedent in historic times" that will cause "changes in climate patterns that are likely to have enormous impacts on global civilization."

The media have been quick to jump on these and other statements as evidence of a tremendous threat from rising global temperatures. But many scientists studying the problem complain that journalists have seized on the extremes in this debate, as in many others, making it seem as though most "right-thinking" researchers agree on the severity of global warming, and that those who don't are simply apologists for industry. Scientists willing to express their "greenhouse anxiety" publicly have attracted almost adulatory attention from environmentalists and the press.

But by examining global warming more closely, we can see what the real risks are and who is benefiting by blowing certain risks out of proportion.

Global warming first hit the newsstands in 1987, which had one of the hottest summers on record. We were primed to hear about heat. Newspapers and television told us that we were heating up the earth's atmosphere by driving our cars and running our factories — in other words, by burning oil and coal, which creates carbon dioxide. Other man-made gases such as methane were also culprits. Scientists predicted that at the current rates at which we were creating carbon dioxide, the average temperature of the world would increase half a degree Fahrenheit each decade, rising four degrees Fahrenheit by 2050 and nine degrees by the year 2100.

Would this temperature change make much difference? Vice President Gore says that even a slight temperature shift could be catastrophic. He points out that when the global temperature was only six degrees Celsius lower than it is today, New York City was under a kilometer of ice. That slightly lower temperature meant a mini-ice age.

That's pretty scary. If a small temperature change makes such a difference, we'd better assess whether that change is really going to happen. Are these predictions of global warming correct?

Scientists use computer models to try to figure out what will happen in the atmosphere over the long term. It's these models that have led to the predictions of the greenhouse effect. The computers have concluded that, given all the variables, man-made carbon dioxide will seriously increase the atmospheric temperature.

However, these computer models don't take into account what has really happened over the past hundred years before making such predictions. During the twentieth century, increases in carbon dioxide emissions into the atmosphere haven't been associated at all with higher temperatures. *Reason* magazine (March 1993) points out that carbon dioxide has increased by 25 percent, while the greenhouse effect has grown only 1 percent. In fact, during the thirty years after World War II, when we were spewing forth carbon dioxide and other greenhouse gases, the world's temperature actually dropped. The National Academy of Science even proclaimed that we were about to enter a new mini-ice age!

It *is* true that overall the average global temperature has risen one degree since 1880 or so. (That post–World War II period was an exception.) But most of that temperature rise occurred before 1940, despite the fact that most of the carbon dioxide increase came *after* 1940 (*Commentary*, July 1993).

How about all the carbon dioxide we've emitted this past decade? The computer estimates tell us that all the greenhouse gases from the 1980s should have led to a half-degree global temperature rise. But the temperature only rose one-tenth of a degree.

Why would people exaggerate something as serious as the greenhouse effect? Climatologist Stephen Schneider explained in *Discover* magazine (October 1989) that scientists have to "capture the public's imagination" in order to get funding. "So," he continued, "we have to offer up scary scenarios, make simplified, dramatic statements, and make little mention of any doubts we may have." By the way, this same scientist is one of the many who warned about the ice age coming in the 1970s. Now he is quoted very frequently on global warming.

Schneider speaks out not to contradict himself but to make a point. As an environmentalist, he uses various pieces of evidence (such as scientific data) to promote a certain lifestyle and value system. However, antienvironmentalists (whom we might call proindustrialists) also use scientific data to promote their values. They draw on the many published, respected studies that contradict parts of the global warming theory. All sides of the issue use what they can find.

Take clouds as an example of the many factors that influence the greenhouse debate. Clouds contribute to the greenhouse effect (warming up the climate) because they hold in heat. (Have you noticed that it's often warmer on a cloudy day than on a clear day?) When we pump carbon dioxide into the sky, the atmosphere heats up. As this happens, seawater evaporates and turns into more clouds. But more clouds also mean that less sunlight gets into the earth's atmosphere, which keeps us cooler. This means that clouds protect us against the catastrophic global warming trends that we hear about.

Another "heat button" affecting the world's temperatures is the growth of cities. Cities mean pavement, and pavement reflects more heat into the atmosphere than soil or ground. Many cities, such as Phoenix, have seen the average temperature in the area rise over time as the city spread. The average increase in Phoenix, reported *Reason* magazine in 1993, has been five degrees. Is that catastrophic global warming, or simply civilization advancing as it always has?

All this hot air over global warming is expensive. Taxpayers spend over $1 billion to pay eighteen federal agencies just to analyze the issue (*St. Petersburg Times*, 16 May 1993). Cooling down our carbon dioxide emissions — which, as we've seen, don't necessarily cause global warming in the first place — would be even more expensive. The Department of Energy says that a 20 percent reduction in carbon dioxide by the year 2000 would mean doubling the price of electricity, tripling oil prices, and quintupling the price of coal. That's only for the United States, which produces 30 percent of the world's greenhouse gases.

As for the rest of the world, developing countries want to use their coal to bring themselves into the twenty-first century. If they're not allowed to do that, they're going to need a lot more help than they're already receiving from the rest of the world to find new energy sources.

What conclusions can we draw? The only things that are clear at this point are that, yes, carbon dioxide emissions do warm the atmosphere, but by how much and to what effect, we still don't know. Which means that it probably doesn't make a lot of sense to panic when you hear the words "global warming" or "greenhouse effect" — at least not yet.

# "THE SKY IS FALLING!"

O r, at least, it's becoming riddled with holes in the all-important ozone layer. Some scientists claim that the world's use of refrigeration emits an unsafe level of CFCs — chlorofluorocarbons — into the atmosphere. Those CFCs, the story goes, are eating into the ozone layer, the "safety blanket" that keeps the sun's cancer-causing ultraviolet rays from killing us all.

So slather yourself with sunscreen, or buy lots of wide-brim hats and wear them all the time. Give up tennis. Don't go to the beach. You're closer to the sun at high altitudes, so don't hike in the mountains. Better yet, don't go outside at all if you want to avoid skin cancer. Turn off your refrigerator and don't use your car's air-conditioning; both deplete the ozone layer and increase your risk.

Is this good advice? Is the sky "falling"? Should we be worried about the ozone layer? What does science have to say?

A review of the scientific evidence leads to these conclusions: Yes, it's a good idea to avoid overusing air-conditioning, but certainly not if you're very hot. Absolutely keep your refrigerator turned *on*. Wear a hat or sunscreen to avoid painful sunburn, but please do go outdoors and enjoy getting some exercise.

What is ozone? It's a form of oxygen that exists in three-atom clusters, and is created when solar ultraviolet rays smash into and split apart molecules of ordinary oxygen. If one of these newly freed oxygen atoms collides with another molecule of ordinary oxygen, they form a new three-atom molecule of ozone. Atmospheric ozone absorbs ultraviolet B rays, which are especially injurious to all living cells.

Scientists have agreed that CFCs destroy ozone. The chlorine in CFCs cuts into the oxygen molecules that make up ozone, allowing ultraviolet rays to pass through to earth. However, ozone is being dissolved and reformed all the time, usually by natural sources. Ozone, scientists tell us, is a renewable resource. Still, every time a volcano erupts or seawater evaporates, ozone is depleted. These sources release far more chlorine into the atmosphere than man-made CFCs. But man-made products don't just *deplete* ozone. Cars, for example, actually increase ozone levels. In smoggy Los Angeles, cars emit enough air pollution to reduce ultraviolet levels by 6 to 9 percent on an average day (*Skeptical Inquirer*, Fall 1994).

But what about the famous "ozone hole" over Antarctica? This "hole" is a thinning of the ozone layer to about one-third its normal depth (at its worst) during certain seasons. Some people fear that CFCs will cause a hole over the Arctic, too, which eventually will spread over populated regions, bringing skin cancer and other radiation-related diseases to the earth's inhabitants. Even worse than skin cancer, though, will be the extinction of organisms lowest on the food chain, such as phytoplankton. With the tiniest food sources gone, the smallest organisms (such as little fish) will die. And on it will go until the food-chain-turned-death-chain reaches humans. Eventually, we, too, would have nothing to eat.

Is this "ozone hole" as serious as it sounds? To begin with, whether the hole is recent or not, it existed before human-generated CFCs were around. Scientists in the 1950s found annual variations in the ozone layer above Antarctica, including what we now call the ozone hole. Ozone depletion is a natural phenomenon in Antarctica.

Is the ozone layer being depleted above the entire world? Doomsayers claim that the ozone hole is worsening every year. However, these people are looking at statistics only from the past fourteen years. Ozone levels regularly fluctuate around the world and over time. We can't predict a real trend from only fourteen years of reliable data. According to physicist Dr. S. Fred Singer, ozone fluctuates as much as 40 percent over the seasons of the year. The normal cycle of sunspots, which lasts eleven years, also continues to the up-and-down of ozone levels. That's because when there are sunspots, the spectrum of solar radiation is best for producing additional ozone. As Dr. Singer put it, drawing conclusions about long-term ozone changes from a single decade "is like observing temperatures for one season and judging whether climate has changed over the long term" (*Garbage* magazine, September–October 1993).

It's also not necessarily true that less ozone in the sky means more UV rays on the ground. Despite the fact that the northern hemisphere's ozone blanket is a bit thinner during the springtime, no one has been able to find additional UV rays on the ground during those times. In fact, *Nature* magazine reported on 28 September 1989 that scientists even found a *decrease* in UV rays between 1968 and 1982, when ozone levels were low.

Moreover, there are no research studies linking skin cancer, cataracts, and the other alleged problems to increased UV radiation from ozone loss. Then why, you might ask, is skin cancer increasing? Take your gaze down from the sky and look around at our world. Through the '60s, '70s, and '80s (and somewhat still in the '90s), tans were "in." That wasn't the case before the '60s. Sunbathing — in skimpier bathing suits — became popular. The southwest United States (known as the Sunbelt) drew millions of people to build cities in the hot, sun-drenched desert. And most of these people are Caucasians, thought to be more susceptible to the dangers of ultraviolet radiation. More people are getting skin cancer because more people are in the sun — not because the sun is inherently more dangerous or because there's less ozone.

Don't just take our word for it. In September–October 1993, the magazine *Garbage*, which leans heavily toward the side of environmentalists, studied the ozone issue and drew some conclusions that probably led to a few subscription cancellations by ardent environmentalists. The magazine concluded, "There is currently no 'crisis,' nor any documented threat to human health," from the ozone layer. *Garbage* found that "(a) the so-called ozone hole is an ephemeral disturbance over a mostly unpopulated area; (b) ozone thinning over populated latitudes, if it exists, is within the range of normal fluctuation and is seasonal; (c) no documentation exists to prove a sustained increase in UV-B radiation at ground level. . . ."

But wait. This is difficult reading, and it's a beautiful sunny day outside. It's time to put on shorts and a tank top, and go "catch some rays. . . ." Don't be afraid to join us, but do put on sunscreen.

# DEATH BY DIOXIN?

**D**ioxin has been blamed for fetal deformities, miscarriages, lung cancer, liver cancer, severe rashes, depression, numbness, and memory loss. Supposedly it's in the fish, meat, and dairy products we eat. In fact, dioxin was recently named in a two-thousand-page Environmental Protection Agency report as a leading candidate in causing cancer. We suspected all along that dioxin caused serious problems — we saw this in Vietnam veterans exposed to Agent Orange, which contains dioxin — but now it's official.

Is dioxin as bad as people say? What are the *real* dangers versus the hype?

Dioxin is nearly everywhere, though less so now than twenty years ago. Virtually all of us in industrialized society have some dioxin in our bodies. Dioxin enters our food supply from a variety of sources. It is emitted during the manufacture of chlorine and chlorinated compounds and when industrial plants burn municipal and medical waste that contains chlorine. It also is associated with the bleaching of wood pulp during paper manufacturing. The dioxin gets into the groundwater and then ends up in the ocean, where it contaminates fish, especially near the coasts of big cities. Dioxin ends up in milk and meat through a similar process. The toxic groundwater soaks into the soil, which produces "toxic" grass. When cows eat grass containing dioxin, the chemical settles in their fatty substances, which include milk as well as meat.

When humans ingest dioxin, it also accumulates in the body's fatty tissue. Someone exposed to a lot of dioxin, such as some Vietnam veterans with respect to Agent Orange, might not see the effects of dioxin for years after the exposure. Losing weight can make dioxin come forward because the ratio of fat (and dioxin) to overall body weight drops. In this sense, because dioxin accumulates, even tiny doses eventually can be fatal.

The evidence that dioxin causes cancer is sufficiently strong to make the EPA ask industrial polluters to follow stricter guidelines on dioxin. Although the EPA has already placed over thirty different restrictions on dioxin — from its use in manufacturing to herbicides — it wants additional safeguards.

*However . . .*

The EPA also found that the worst effects of dioxin require at least ten to one hundred times the amount that most of us receive in our food (*Los Angeles Times*, 12 September 1994). In fact, the EPA believes that the level of dioxin in people has been declining in recent years. The EPA isn't advising Americans to change what we eat. Nor did the EPA go so far as to name dioxin a "known carcinogen." It called dioxin a "probable" but weak carcinogen. Only animal studies have been conducted so far, and as we've seen, we can't always generalize from animal studies to humans. As William Farland, director of the Office of Health and Environmental Assessment for EPA, put it, there is a "data gap" in scientists' understanding of dioxin in foods.

The public and some scientists have long considered dioxin to be one of the strongest artificial carcinogens. Dioxin was the chemical that caused the terror behind the Love Canal and Times Beach crises. More recently, though, public officials have wondered if we didn't overreact to the dioxin scare. Vernon Houk, director of the Center for Environmental Health at the Centers for Disease Control, was responsible for the 1982 evacuation of Times Beach, Missouri, when oil contaminated with dioxin spread through the streets. Eight years after the crisis, Mr. Houk said that because dioxin has been found to be only a "weak carcinogen" — as confirmed even more by the EPA in 1994 — he wouldn't order the evacuation if the same crisis arose again. Several studies came to similar conclusions about Love Canal (New York) and even about Agent Orange.

The story of one reporter illustrates how dioxin fears might be overblown. Pulitzer Prize–winning journalist Jon Franklin investigated the dioxin controversy in 1982 while writing an article on Agent Orange. Franklin grew up as a liberal activist protesting against chemical companies. He admitted that his approach to the article was characterized less by journalistic objectivity than by "the righteous fervor that is the armor of the crusading reporter." However, by the end of his investigation, Franklin found no solid medical evidence of dioxin leading to fetal abnormalities and cancers. He concluded that the Agent Orange story, and the accompanying fears about dioxin spread by the mass media, were myths created by antiwar activists.

Dioxin *is* deadly, so we can thank the government for regulating it so strongly and effectively. The dioxin story is an example of a government program working right: as soon as dioxin was identified as a problem, its use was restricted, and we now carry less of it in our bodies than we used to. For the vast majority of people, dioxin is not really a threat. As Gregg Easterbrook wrote in *Newsweek* magazine (as quoted from the *Los Angeles Times*, 11 September 1994), "[Environmental protection] is one public policy and technology area where programs are successful . . . something to be optimistic about."

# ELECTROMAGNETIC FIELDS: A FIELD OF DREAMS?

Y ou're looking for a new place to live. A real estate agent has found you a charming house — lots of light, great location, good price. You're looking through the house, thinking that this is "the one." Then you glance out of one of the pretty windows and see a snarl of electrical utility wires anchored into a hefty T-shaped transformer. It's within twelve feet of the wall.

You pale a bit. Didn't the newspaper recently say something about electromagnetic fields from these transformers causing cancer? Or was it Alzheimer's disease? You remember: it was both.

You turn to the agent. "Uh . . . the house is nice, but. . . ." You wonder if this whole story about electromagnetic fields is just a myth. You hate to give up this house. But it's better to be safe than sorry, right? Nevertheless, you feel silly about being so worried. "It's nice, but not exactly what I was looking for. Thanks anyway." You're dejected.

On your way home — to your very boring, tiny, dark apartment with no power transformers anywhere near — you stop by the library to investigate the "truth" behind electromagnetic fields. Did you just give up that great place in vain? Maybe it's not too late to change your mind once you know the truth about the health effects of living near power lines.

You find stories about electromagnetic fields, or EMFs, as scientists call them, that appeared in newspapers and magazines during the summer of 1994. Scientific studies from Finland and Los Angeles found that EMFs "could play an important role" (whatever that means, you grumble) in Alzheimer's disease. EMFs have also been linked to leukemia, brain tumors, and breast cancer. Earlier studies found that children living close to high-voltage electrical wires have leukemia at 2.5 times the national average (*Los*

*Angeles Times,* 11 February 1991). A California couple sued their local electric company because, they said, their daughter got two types of rare cancer
from electromagnetic fields — while she was in the uterus.

Good thing you're not going to live next to that power transformer.

What seems to happen when people are exposed to EMFs, the scientists
say, is a disruption at the cellular level. Calcium ions in the cells vibrate with
the electromagnetic waves, and then the cells can't communicate with each
other. As Cedric Garland, an epidemiologist and expert in public health,
put it in an article in the *Los Angeles Times* (30 May 1991), "Intercellular
communication is what prevents cancer. When it's disrupted, a precondi-
tion of cancer is thus created." EMFs can also cause tiny parts of brain cells
to "tangle," which characterizes Alzheimer's disease.

Just as you're about to leave, satisfied with yourself for the decision you've
made, a few words on a magazine page catch your eye: EMFs are also found
in sewing machines. Hair dryers. Electric blankets. Home computers. Television sets. Electric alarm clocks. Cellular phones. Stereos. All electrical
home appliances. . . . EMFs are everywhere!

Moreover, it turns out that the electromagnetic fields emanating from
power lines are not very strong. EMFs are measured in gauss; nearby power
lines radiate 5 to 40 milligauss (thousands of gauss). But stand a foot away
from many home appliances, and the milligauss will measure from as little
as 1 milligauss — to as many as 280 milligauss. Electric can openers, by the
way, emit the most milligauss among common kitchen appliances. You also
learn that magnetic fields diminish sharply with distance.

You sit back down. Not only are EMFs part of our technological society
everywhere we go, but the "link" between EMFs and cancer isn't necessarily proven. An important study in Denver found a relationship between types
of wiring in high-power lines and leukemia — but a follow-up study, which
measured the EMF level inside the homes in that same area, found the exact
opposite: a weaker association between higher EMF in the home and
leukemia rates. Other studies, such as one done at the University of Southern California in the early 1990s, found no significant increase in leukemia
in children due to residential power line exposure. And some highly respected scientists, from research universities such as Harvard, challenge the
whole idea of links between EMFs and cancer.

You look up from your reading. It seems that electromagnetic fields are
ubiquitous. They're the price of living in a society with electricity, which
has brought infinitely more benefit than harm. It also seems that scientists
just aren't clear yet whether residential power lines emit enough EMFs to
be dangerous. Also, there are different types of lines to take into account:

the high-voltage lines that bring electricity across the country, and the lower-voltage lines found in all residential neighborhoods. Living under one of those high-voltage transitional lines might not be good for your health. But as for the little transformer outside the window of that great house. . . .

If living next to power lines caused cancer, lots more people probably would have cancer, because most of us live near some sort of power line. For people who are still concerned about EMFs, utility companies can measure the electromagnetic field in an area. You stand up to leave the library, thinking about the situation. Maybe you'll ask the utility company to measure the EMFs after you move into the house — or maybe you won't.

# NUKING THE MUSHROOM CLOUD OF FEAR

**M**any people remember the tragic and deadly accident at the Chernobyl nuclear power plant in the former Soviet Union. The images of children wasting away and later dying are etched in our minds. Others remember the less-serious, but nonetheless frightening, 1979 accident at the nuclear power plant at Three Mile Island in Pennsylvania. In light of these mishaps, it makes sense that we're afraid of nuclear power plants. There is enough radiation stored in only one of these plants to decimate the globe. A nuclear power plant meltdown, like the one in Chernobyl in 1986, can wreak dramatic human and environmental destruction whose effects endure for generations.

Thousands of protesters gather at nuclear plants across the globe and shout: "No nukes! No nukes! No nukes!" No one wants a nuclear power plant in their state, much less their city. The Three Mile Island disaster filled headlines for weeks, fueling our fears of nuclear energy. "Three Mile Island: Notes from a Nightmare," read a *New York Times* headline. The evening news screamed that our nuclear power plants are already aging and that we could be facing a nuclear disaster. Now, almost two decades after Three Mile Island, the memory is charged with fear. Could another nuclear accident — or something worse — happen again?

Even the less politically active among us believe we probably shouldn't be building nuclear power plants. Nothing is foolproof, and a nuclear disaster raises the word *disaster* to new heights. Millions would die; groundwater would become radioactive. Radioactivity would be released into the atmosphere, leading to higher rates of skin cancer, birth defects, leukemia, you name it. Agricultural soil would become contaminated. And the contamination would render the area uninhabitable for decades, perhaps centuries.

How dangerous is it really to develop nuclear energy today? To balance our view of nuclear energy, we should try to open our minds and look beyond doomsday scenarios. Scientists, who know more about the risks of nuclear energy than we do, believe that we *should* develop this technology. They think that while nuclear energy is one of the most potentially destructive technologies, it can be handled safely. Nuclear energy potentially is one of the most beneficial technologies in our world today. Let's look at why we fear nuclear energy to see how well founded our fears actually are.

The first time many of us became aware of the risks of nuclear power was the Three Mile Island crisis. Since then, planning and construction of new nuclear power plants in the United States have come to a virtual halt, largely because of public fears. Polls show that in 1971, eight years before Three Mile Island, 58 percent of Americans were willing to have a nuclear power plant in their own towns. In 1980, the year after Three Mile Island, only 28 percent were willing, and 63 percent were opposed.

Many studies have traced public fears of nuclear energy to media coverage starting with Three Mile Island. The more negative and controversial the coverage of nuclear energy by the media, the higher the public's fear. By now it's been documented in dozens of studies that public concern about any new technology is directly related to the amount of media coverage that technology receives.

The media covered the Three Mile Island crisis as though there had been mass destruction on a global level. But do you realize that no one died as a result of the Three Mile Island crisis? Moreover, independent researchers have found no solid evidence of increased cancer in the area years after the incident. As David Shaw of the *Los Angeles Times* (13 September 1994) put it in an excellent series of articles on fear, risk, and the media, "Residents probably put themselves at greater risk driving away from Three Mile Island than they would have by staying." He was referring to the everyday risk of driving an automobile, which is far higher but less publicized than many smaller but highly publicized risks, such as a nuclear meltdown.

The government even created a special task force to examine this media coverage. Their conclusion? Journalists "knew shockingly little about nuclear power and compounded their ignorance by focusing too narrowly on worst-case scenarios," said David Rubin, who headed the task force, in the *Los Angeles Times* (September 13, 1994). In fact, the task force went so far as to say, "To a reader or viewer trying to decide whether to pack his bags and run [from Three Mile Island], radiation reports in the media were often as useless as a baseball score of 6–4 that neglected to mention which teams had played."

Pretty scathing. This poor coverage is especially shameful considering that the Three Mile Island incident is actually an example of a nuclear power plant working. The shut-down system worked. The power station turned off. Disaster was averted by the systems set in place to prevent it. And the government drastically modified regulations to prevent another, similar problem.

As a result of such media coverage, many people rank nuclear power as the number-one hazard in our times. However, scientists rank it much lower on the list, after crime, swimming, driving, and other risks that are statistically far more common. Lost amid the coverage of the Chernobyl disaster was another crucial fact: The type of reactor that experienced problems at Chernobyl exists only in the former Soviet Union. Western nations prohibit such dangerously designed plants.

If the vast majority of scientists feel that nuclear power is safe, why are we still so afraid of it? This issue epitomizes many of the ways in which we're scaring ourselves to death. It's the type of issue that is usually covered poorly by the media — highly technical and potentially very sensational. It's an issue that is easily manipulated by various interest groups for political purposes. Nuclear energy is the issue that launched the environmental movement, which often uses scare tactics to gain support.

Another reason we're so afraid of nuclear energy is that the potential risks are beyond our personal control. We might choose to go skydiving, willingly taking on such a high risk, but we don't want to be subject to potentially deadly mistakes made by scientists and engineers. Also, radiation is invisible, and nothing is scarier than the invisible. Despite its invisibility, radiation is one of the deadliest and most horrifying threats in our modern age. It causes slow, painful death; it gives birth to terrifying deformities, and it has the potential for large-scale destruction.

Moreover, we're often afraid of new technologies simply because they're new. People were frightened of electricity, of cars, and steam engines when each of these technologies was first introduced. It's the same with nuclear power. But nuclear energy could provide a solution to other risks such as greenhouse gases warming our atmosphere. Nuclear energy is "cleaner" than coal, for example, which causes serious pollution problems. Nuclear energy releases far less carbon dioxide into the atmosphere. Nuclear power could also help us shift the balance of political power away from dependency on those volatile Middle Eastern nations that produce most of the world's oil. Oil provides almost 50 percent of the entire world's fuel; half of the oil consumed in the United States comes from foreign countries. If we no longer needed so much foreign oil, we would have much less reason to become entangled in foreign nations' problems simply because they had a natural resource vital to our economy.

Experts also recognize that our supply of conventional, nonrenewable fuels such as coal, oil, and wood is limited, and not nearly big enough to sustain the current rates of development. In fact, some predict widespread oil and gas shortages by the end of the century. Nuclear energy could help solve that problem. Energy produced by nuclear fusion, which scientists have not yet figured out how to harness, could solve the world's energy problems for thousands of years. Experts say it will take another ten to twenty years before commercial nuclear fusion plants are ready to come on line — largely because we are so careful to install extensive safety features in the plants.

Since scientists first harnessed the power of nuclear fission, nuclear energy has emerged as a major source for electric energy around the world. At the end of 1989, the world had 416 operating nuclear power plants, which generated 17 percent of global electricity. The United States has the most plants of any country in the world: 108 in operation, providing almost 20 percent of the electrical energy (*Grolier's Multimedia Encyclopedia*, 1993).

Nuclear power is one solution. All solutions carry risks — everything in life carries risks — but in this case it seems that the benefits far outweigh the potential harm, thanks to the safeguards we have put in place.

# GO FISH

We've been told that fish is one of the healthiest choices on the menu. It's "brain food," our mothers and doctors say. Eating fish will make you smart.

Well, if eating fish has made us smart, is it now time to use our brains and avoid eating fish? That's what the National Academy of Science tells us, not to mention news headlines around the country. According to them, our fish supply has been contaminated by both bacteria and chemical pollutants. Let's examine the arguments for avoiding fish, then compare them with the benefits of including fish in our diets and see which side comes swimming to the surface.

The first and scariest argument against eating fish is chemical contamination. In 1991, the National Academy of Sciences warned that seafood is hazardous to our health. Fish and shellfish carry environmental toxins such as methyl mercury, polychlorinated biphenyl, dioxin, and the infamous DDT. Most industrialized nations have banned the use of some of these chemicals, such as DDT, but we used enough of them in previous decades that some of them are still present in the world's water supply. And when it rains, dioxin from the smokestacks of industrial plants returns to our groundwater, where it contaminates the fish.

The most chemically contaminated fish in the United States, says the Academy, are found in the Great Lakes, inland waterways, and coastal bays and estuaries. That sounds like nearly everywhere we can fish in this country — except maybe Hawaii. The Academy thinks that about 75 out of every 1 million consumers are at risk of cancer from eating fish. That's far above the usual safety standard set by the government for issuing cancer warnings. The usual "alert" standard is only 1 in 1 million.

These risk estimates have been supported by scientific studies. Babies born to women who eat PCB-contaminated fish from the Great Lakes have lower birth weight and smaller heads. Some of these babies also have neurological problems.

So far, the outlook isn't good for our consumption of fish, thanks to the way we have allowed our use of pesticides and other chemicals to contaminate our fishing waters. Unfortunately the story doesn't improve much when we look at bacterial contamination of seafood.

About sixty thousand people become sick from seafood poisoning each year (*Los Angeles Times*, 18 February 1994). Most become ill after eating raw shellfish. Fin fish also carry potentially dangerous bacteria, but these fish are usually cooked, killing the bacteria before it can make us sick. One federal risk assessment study, reported in the *Los Angeles Times* on 31 January 1994, found that 1 out of every 1,000 servings of raw oysters, clams, or mussels contains lethal levels of dangerous bacteria.

Oysters have been shown to cause *Vibrio vulnificus*, a serious bacterial infection that usually leads to death. A California man won a million-dollar settlement after coming down with this infection, which resulted in severe muscle and bone damage. According to the Centers for Disease Control, Louisiana oysters in just one month alone — November 1993 — caused 180 cases of diarrhea, vomiting, nausea, cramps, and fever.

California now requires supermarkets and restaurants to post warning signs if they sell or serve oysters caught in the Gulf of Mexico. California even wants to go a step further and warn the entire public to avoid eating any raw shellfish at all. Why? The FDA only inspects seafood plants every three to five years, and the budget for seafood inspections is not nearly enough to inspect most seafood. A great deal of hazardous seafood, especially shellfish, can easily slip through the holes in the net of regulations and inspection.

Quite understandably, all of these problems have eroded public confidence in seafood. Since the late 1980s seafood sales have declined because the public is concerned about the safety of the food.

Now for the crucial question: Should *you* stop eating seafood? In spite of all the stories, studies, and doomsaying reported above, the answer is no.

One way we measure the potential danger of a particular type of food is by looking at how many people get sick out of how many people are served that food. The *Los Angeles Times* (31 January 1994) reports that the infection rate for *all* seafood, including raw shellfish, is about 1 out of every 250,000 servings. That's ten times safer than chicken, which makes one of us sick out of every 25,000 servings. Also, the U.S. Food and Drug Administration recently set new, stricter rules on seafood processing plants. The risk is decreasing every day.

Moreover, the risk of becoming ill by eating cooked fin fish — the tuna, swordfish, bass, catfish, and so forth that most of us think of when we think "seafood" — has always been very low. The cooking process kills most, if not all, harmful bacteria. If you avoid raw shellfish, you reduce your risk even further.

Think about the overall population of fish-eaters in the United States. Americans eat fifteen pounds of seafood per person per year, on average. Out of all that, only sixty thousand people develop gastroenteritis (food poisoning) from seafood. That's 1 in 216,666 servings. According to these odds, if you ate seafood at every single meal of your life, you could live to age seventy-two before you became ill from seafood.

Regarding the risk of chemical contamination, it's true that our fish does sometimes contain dioxin, DDT, and other harmful chemicals. However, the levels of these chemicals are usually far below those considered dangerous, and won't harm you unless you eat a lot of fish — virtually for your entire diet — and unless that fish comes from highly contaminated regions, such as the Great Lakes.

So, the odds of getting sick from seafood aren't high enough to be overly concerned about, particularly if you avoid raw shellfish and eat a varied diet. And the risks really pale when you consider the exceptional health benefits of fish. Fish provides excellent protein and is low in fat. It's also a great source of vitamins, including Vitamin E. Fish truly is "brain food" in many ways: It makes you smart, and you're smart to eat it.

# THE SPERM, THE EGG, AND THE INDUSTRIAL
# REVOLUTION

**P**enises are shrinking!" "Sperm can't swim as fast as they used to!" "Women's eggs are malfunctioning!" "Ovaries can't ovulate!" Biologists are becoming good headline writers for the tabloids. They claim that the chemicals and pesticides we have developed to make our lives safer and more comfortable are actually causing abnormalities in our reproductive systems that are making us less fertile as a species.

This topic is a headline-grabber like few others. It focuses on our sexuality and on our ability to reproduce, both of which are basic sources of self-esteem and identity. A single headline warning us that we might not be able to have children, or that penises are shrinking, ovaries can't ovulate, and so on, is enough to scare us very seriously.

Fortunately, by taking a critical look at the story behind the headlines, we can rest a bit more comfortably.

The headlines were drawn from a highly disputed study, published in 1992, conducted internationally by Danish researchers, who identified a noticeably lower sperm count among men over the past fifty years. The alleged cause is environmental pollution. An American biologist took this study to Congress with these fighting words: "Every man sitting in this room today is half the man his grandfather was. And the question is, are our children going to be half the men we are?" (*Los Angeles Times*, 3 October 1994).

Doomsayers have coupled the results of this study with what seems to be an increase in other reproductive problems. Testicular and prostate cancer have doubled among men in industrialized countries. Breast cancer and endometriosis have sped up among women. And infertility seems to be a growing problem in both sexes.

What's their explanation? Industrial pollution is responsible for the increase in reproductive disorders, according to these doomsayers. Industrial chemicals, such as pesticides, can actually act like sex hormones, imitating estrogen or stopping testosterone development in its tracks. That's part of why these chemicals are effective as pesticides.

However — and this is a big "however" — let's take a deep breath and look critically at all of these allegations. You'll see that they're unfounded, or at the very least that there is far too little reliable research from which to draw these conclusions.

First, the one crucial study, conducted by the Danish researchers, is highly disputed by other scientists. However, the media never reported how and why it was so disputed. It's important to remember that most journalists are trained only to *report* the news. They're generally not trained to evaluate the scientific validity of studies. The *Los Angeles Times* (13 September 1994) once published a joke that if scientist John Doe claimed that Newton, Galileo, and Einstein were wrong about the world being round, newspaper reporters would probably report Doe's findings. The media will report a study claiming low sperm count because it's "news" (not to mention being a great headline-grabber), but they won't be able to evaluate the validity of that study. The lesson here: Always analyze news stories critically.

Second, look at the reported increase in prostate cancer, testicular cancer, breast cancer, and endometriosis. All of these can be explained by factors other than industrial pollution. People live longer, and thus have more years in which to develop cancer. Fifty years ago, people died around age sixty. Now we live to be almost eighty, on average. Prostate, testicular, and breast cancer are largely diseases of older men and women. The number of people with cancer is growing at least in part because our population is aging.

The increase in cases of endometriosis can be explained by a factor that is much more likely to be the real culprit than industrial pollution: the sexual revolution. The incidence of sexually transmitted diseases and a variety of sexual infections is growing right along with the increase in sexual activity. Endometriosis has been linked to these infections because, left untreated, such infections can lead to endometriosis. This seems to be a more likely cause than industrial pollution. (It is also, of course, a preventable cause. Safe sex and regular visits to the doctor can prevent most cases of endometriosis. But that's good news, and the media doesn't report good news nearly as frequently as bad news.)

Animal studies have indeed shown a link between chemically contaminated fish and reproductive disorders. Animals that are fed high levels of chemicals such as dioxin and DDT often produce offspring with deformed or malfunctioning sexual organs, some of them even having both ovaries and testicles.

Do the kinds of pesticides that might cling to fruit and vegetables or hide in the fatty tissue of beef mimic hormones so that our real hormones don't work? The reality is that we ingest estrogen and other hormones from the environment all the time. We consume tons of "natural" estrogen and estrogen inhibitors in fruits and vegetables. These compounds, called flavonoids, do us no harm. Neither do other forms of naturally occurring external estrogen that we ingest. Our body's natural hormonal resources are hundreds of times stronger than any estrogen-pretender in pesticides.

Some argue that environmentalists and others who oppose pesticides are promoting this issue as a way to scare people and politicians into banning pesticides altogether. Threatening someone's identity as a reproductive being can be an effective tactic.

And it turns out that the sperm level in men *has* declined during the last fifty years. On average, men today have 66 million sperm per milliliter of semen. That's down from 113 million just after World War II, but still quite a lot. Most scientists agree that 20 million sperm per milliliter of semen — less than one-third the current average — are adequate for normal reproduction (*Sierra*, March–April 1993).

So what *is* responsible for the lower sperm count over the past fifty years? Hot tubs? Tight underwear? Marijuana? All have been called culprits. The jury is still out on this question. But the EPA and scientists embroiled in this debate do agree on one thing: The best way to avoid this particular risk is for pregnant women not to eat too many fats, which harbor pesticide residues more than other food substances. For most people, reducing the amount of fat in their diet is good advice regardless of whether these reproductive risks are real or not.

# CONCLUSION

# WHO LOSES? WHO WINS?

There is nothing to fear but fear itself.

— Franklin Delano Roosevelt

**A**s we've seen, scaring ourselves to death is itself a scary proposition. Not only can our fears be far worse than the things we're afraid of, but *the fears themselves* actually can harm us more. Who loses in the overhyping of "risks" today? *You do.* Who wins? The lawyers, the media, politicians, regulators, special interest groups. . . .

## HOW DO YOU LOSE?

Although it does not carry a warning label, our political system may be hazardous to our health.

— Harvey M. Sapolsky, Professor of Public Policy and Organization, Massachusetts Institute of Technology

You lose by putting time, energy, worry, and money into risks that aren't necessarily serious. Do you really need BGH-free milk or organic produce — at up to twice the price? Should you really drive across the country to avoid taking that airplane flight? Is it worth a sleepless night tossing and turning, worrying that you could contract a mystery virus that baffles scientists? Should you feel conflicted when you turn on a light, knowing that some of the energy comes from nuclear power? Are you comfortable putting tax dollars into expensive risk assessment to check for electromagnetic fields or asbestos in schools where the parents' voices seem louder than those of scientists?

We lose even more seriously by giving attention to negligible (but dramatic) risks at the expense of real risks. There *are* real risks in our world. Risk analyst Harvey Sapolsky laments that our political system as well as the media "hunts small risks ruthlessly while permitting bigger ones to exist relatively unmolested. It invests billions, seeking unobtainable safety while failing to provide the resources necessary to protect our future. Hardly anyone is saved by the collective mania with risk; many may be harmed by what goes undone."

We saw how New York City residents became hysterical about the risk of asbestos in the schools. It didn't matter that scientists found asbestos levels to be "minuscule" — between 10,000 to 100,000 times lower than the asbestos levels that gave lung cancer to asbestos workers. The government had to respond anyway, putting millions of dollars into alleviating a tiny risk. Could there have been a better use of that money? How about prenatal care, other preventive services, housing, schools, highway safety, or school lunches? What else can you think of?

When we scare ourselves to death, real risks might not get noticed. Infinitely more likely to cause harm than the Ebola virus, for instance, is the appalling lack of basic vaccinations in inner-city children. Or the rapid rise in tuberculosis, first seen in immigrants and now spreading among the general population. Or drunk drivers swerving from lane to lane late on a Saturday night. Or even the backyard swimming pool. None of these risks receive extensive coverage, but they are far more deadly.

In 1987, the Environmental Protection Agency admitted that "overall, EPA's priorities appear more closely aligned with public opinion than with our estimated risks." This is frightening because as taxpayers we pay for the scientists at the EPA to tell *us* what is safe or dangerous and to create policies and regulations to protect us.

In other words, our leaders aren't leading but following. Are we the blind leading the blind? Who *is* leading? Who tells us what's really dangerous and important?

It's not always politicians. While it's gratifying when politicians are sensitive to public opinion, sometimes they use public fears for their own agendas. David Shaw of the *Los Angeles Times* (13 September 1994) drew some damning conclusions from politicians' hypersensitivity to public concerns about risks: "To get reelected, most politicians pass laws and fund programs that address their constituents' fears rather than trying to persuade the body politic that common sense and medical research clearly demonstrate that a particular 'risk' is virtually no risk at all."

All of this means that we're putting money into the wrong places. Biochemist Dr. Bruce Ames puts "scaring ourselves to death" in dollar terms. He thinks we're hurting ourselves by putting media attention and research money in the wrong places. For example, he points out that the Environmental Protection Agency's regulations cost about 2 percent of the United States' Gross National Product — or hundreds of billions of dollars. The price we pay is $50 billion for each life saved through those regulations. On the other hand, "You could give that money to the Highway Department and save a life for, say, $300,000, [by] improving a freeway. If you put the money into basic research, you're probably saving a life for $100,000. . . . With all the scare stories, people don't know what's important anymore."

Another tragedy that comes with scaring ourselves to death is losing good products because of fears that aren't valid. The case of Bendectin, a medication for morning sickness, is a good example. In his book *Galileo's Revenge: Junk Science in the Courtroom*, legal analyst Peter Huber tells the story of how the unfounded claims that this over-the-counter drug caused birth defects caused it to be pulled off the market, when actually it was far more helpful than harmful.

As Hubert tells it, the Bendectin scare was based on "scientific evidence" put forth more by *lawyers* and the tabloid press than by serious medical researchers. The *National Enquirer* ran the story and used this overblown language: "Untold thousands of babies are being born with hideous birth defects . . . several thousand tragically deformed infants in the U.S. alone. . . . a monstrous scandal . . . far worse than the thalidomide horror." The tabloid called the drug Bendectin a "vicious, body-twisting crippler."

What did scientists have to say about the Bendectin scare? Though not a single scientific study had proved the alleged link with birth defects, scientists couldn't get a word in edgewise in this debate. The media were more interested in the sensationalism of the birth defect connection. Bendectin was pulled off the market.

Medical science did have a chance, later, to report on the negative effects of the *loss* of Bendectin. The *Journal of the American Medical Association* reported some problems as a result of Bendectin's *absence*: "a two-fold increase in hospitalizations caused by severe nausea and vomiting in pregnancy since the disappearance of Bendectin. . . ." Women who needed a drug like Bendectin had "severe nausea and vomiting [that] can eventually cause dehydration and acidosis, which threaten the health of the mother and the fetus. . . . Severe cases have led to serious maternal deficiencies and nerve damage. Birth defects may well increase."

With the *loss* of Bendectin — which was driven from the market because of unfounded claims of a link with birth defects — real birth defects were expected to increase. Ironic, isn't it? Young families were the losers when our society scared itself to death.

## WHO WINS?

The risk need not even be real. All that's necessary is a modicum of uncertainty that lawyers can spin into a class-action suit far more profitable for them than for the plaintiffs. . . . Risk inflation of this sort is the true hazard to our health.
—Robert Scheer, writer and social commentator

Certainly the lawyers win. The "Superfund" controversy is a perfect example. The Superfund project was an ambitious, politically charged project to clean up many toxic waste dumps around the country. Many critics of the project believed that the "risks" posed by the toxic waste sites were negligible, but special interests won out. Expenses for cleaning up the Superfund toxic waste sites reached $13.5 billion. Of this amount, 25 percent — almost $3.5 billion — went to lawyers. Was it worth it? Were the Superfund sites cleaned up? Unfortunately, no. In the end only 15 percent of the sites were cleaned. It's the *lawyers* who "cleaned up."

Dozens of huge legal settlements and awards have been made for claims that are very suspect scientifically but that have "scare appeal." Alcolac, Inc., a manufacturer of soaps and cosmetics, was forced to pay $49 million to people whose immune systems were supposedly damaged by the soap plant's pollution. Little if any scientific evidence supported their claims, but they won anyway. The dioxin chemical spill at Times Beach yielded $14.5 million for two defendants, and another dioxin case gave $22 million to the plaintiff — even though the dioxin exposure hadn't been scientifically proven to have caused any illness whatsoever. And so on. In this climate of scaring ourselves to death, unfounded lawsuits tie up our courts and bring big payoffs to lawyers.

Regulators also win from the current climate of fear. While most regulation has been beneficial to our society, some is driven by irrational fears (and sometimes the regulators are in that driver's seat). Overregulation can become more burdensome than helpful to us, while providing lucrative employment for the regulators. Mother Teresa wanted to open an orphanage in New York City, but she couldn't afford to build the elevator required by law. She and her Sisters of Charity were perfectly happy walking up the flights of stairs, but the city just wouldn't allow it. So Mother Teresa couldn't come to New York.

Who else wins? We can't forget the politicians. They regularly play on our fears. Remember George Bush's Willie Horton advertisement? He was playing on our fear of crime. Governor Pete Wilson of California also campaigned on the crime issue, building people's fears of carjacking, drive-by shootings, and more — even though overall, violent crime had dropped in California. (His slogans were "tough on crime" and "three strikes and you're out," promising to keep repeat offenders behind bars.) Suburbanites, who lived in areas where crime was lowest, were the voters who elected this governor. Similar political campaigns have taken place across the United States, exploiting media-hyped fears.

Special interest groups are also winners when we become scared to death. For example, by scaring heterosexuals about AIDS, activists ensure that research funding for AIDS increases. Women's groups do the same for breast cancer. While the causes are often valid, the means of garnering support is often the use of scare tactics.

Every day we encounter media hype, regulations, lawsuits, policies, and public and personal fears. But rather than being the victims of fears that someone else defines, we can analyze the alleged risks intelligently and come to our own conclusions. We can stop being the pawns of special interest groups, lawyers, or politicians.

The next time you encounter a scare story, try to determine "who wins." Is it the gun lobby (playing up fears of crime)? Environmentalists? Health food entrepreneurs? Then think about how *you* can win by clearly understanding the particular risk at hand. How can you intelligently protect yourself and retain a healthy balance in your life? As writer Jonathan Swift wished us, "May you live all the days of your life."